Holistic Health

The Complete Guide to Balanced Living
and Inner Peace

Acknowledgments

Writing Beyond the Body has been a journey of both the heart and the mind, and I am profoundly grateful to all those who have supported me along the way.

First and foremost, I give thanks to God, whose presence, wisdom, and grace have guided me and sustained me throughout this work.

To my family, whose patience, love, and encouragement have been the foundation of my strength, I owe an immeasurable debt of gratitude. Your sacrifices and belief in me have made this endeavor possible.

I am deeply thankful to my colleagues in the medical and academic communities for their insights, critiques, and encouragement. Your contributions helped refine the ideas in this book and gave them greater depth and clarity.

To my students and patients, I am indebted for the lessons you have taught me. Your stories of struggle and resilience, of healing and hope, have been a constant reminder of why this work matters.

To my friends and community, thank you for your prayers, support, and reminders of balance and joy during the long hours of research and writing.

Finally, I dedicate this book to all seekers of truth, health, and wholeness. May these pages inspire you to look beyond the body and embrace the deeper dimensions of life, healing, and spirit.

About the Author

Dr. Inobert Pierre, MD, MBA is a physician, educator, and holistic health advocate with more than three decades of experience in medicine, teaching, and community service. His career has been dedicated not only to clinical practice but also to exploring the deeper connections between mind, body, and spirit.

As a long-time practitioner of yoga and meditation, Dr. Pierre integrates traditional medical knowledge with holistic approaches to healing, emphasizing balance, self-awareness, and preventive care. His work bridges modern science with timeless wisdom, offering practical guidance for those seeking a healthier, more meaningful life.

Through his roles as a doctor, teacher, and mentor, he has inspired countless students, patients, and readers to pursue health in its fullest sense—not merely the absence of disease, but the presence of harmony and wholeness.

Beyond the Body reflects Dr. Pierre's passion for empowering individuals to embrace wellness at every level, inviting readers to look beyond physical health and discover the profound healing potential within.

Table of Contents

Introduction

Years ago, as a young doctor steeped in the practice of allopathy, I found myself at a crossroads. Despite my extensive medical training, I felt something was missing. My patients seemed to improve only temporarily; their symptoms often returned with greater force. One day, a patient asked me if I had ever tried meditation. I laughed it off, skeptical of anything that wasn't grounded in the hard science I had devoted my life to. But her question lingered in my mind. Curious, I decided to explore this unknown path, and what I discovered changed my life forever.

I am Dr. Inobert Pierre, a seasoned allopathy doctor with over twenty years of experience. My journey led me to train in naturopathy, homeopathy, and Ayurveda, and to embrace practices like yoga, meditation, and fasting for over three decades. I have taught these practices for more than ten years, witnessing their transformative power firsthand. My journey from skepticism to advocacy has been profound, and it is this journey that I wish to share with you.

Holistic health is about more than just treating symptoms. It is about achieving a state of complete well-being by integrating mind, body, and spirit. This approach acknowledges that our health is interconnected, and that true healing requires addressing each part of ourselves. It is about living a balanced life in which our physical, mental, and emotional health work in harmony.

In today's fast-paced world, adults face numerous health challenges. Stress is rampant, lifestyle diseases are on the rise, and conventional treatments often fall short. Studies show that stress contributes to 75% of all doctor visits, yet many treatments focus only on symptoms rather than root causes. This is where holistic health steps in, offering a broader view that treats the whole person.

I understand the barriers you may face. Time is limited, information is overwhelming, and skepticism is natural. You may wonder if these practices can fit into your busy life. But I assure you, this book is designed with you in mind. It provides practical, time-efficient solutions that are easy to incorporate into your daily routine.

Throughout this book, we will explore key topics such as exercise, fasting, and mindfulness. These are not just concepts but actionable steps you can take to enhance your well-being. Exercise invigorates the body and mind, fasting offers a reset for our systems, and mindfulness brings clarity and peace. These practices contribute to a holistic approach to health and can be seamlessly integrated into even the busiest of lives.

This book is crafted to be both easy to read and filled with practical tips for improving your health. You will find actionable advice that you can start implementing immediately. Whether it is a quick meditation technique, a simple fasting plan, or an easy exercise routine, these tips are designed to fit into your lifestyle.

My vision for this book is rooted in the belief that true health is achieved through the integration of mind, body, and spirit. I have personally experimented with these practices and know their power. This book is a guide, informed by my own experiences and designed to help you find balance and inner peace.

I invite you to join me on this journey toward holistic health. Let us explore the potential of these practices together. Let us discover the power of integrating mind, body, and spirit in our quest for balanced living. The path to inner peace and well-being is before us, and I am excited to walk it with you.

Chapter 1
The Foundations of Holistic Health

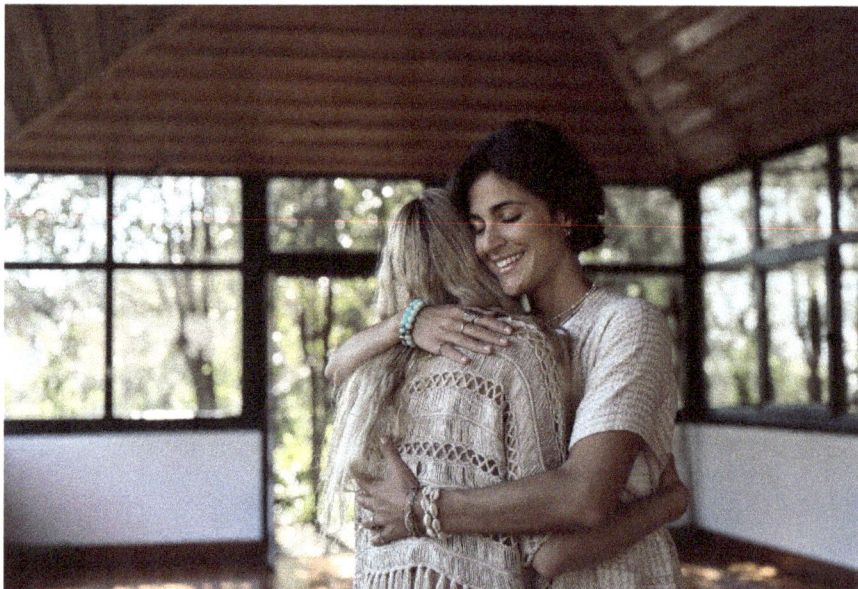

There are moments in life that redefine our understanding of health and well-being. I remember a patient, a young woman burdened with chronic fatigue and anxiety. She had tried everything I prescribed, yet her condition persisted. In a moment of desperation, she asked if there was something beyond the pills and procedures. This encounter sparked a shift in my perspective, prompting me to consider health not just as the absence of disease but as a harmonious balance of the body, mind, and spirit. This revelation set me on a path to explore holistic health, a journey that would transform my practice and my life.

1.1 Understanding the Holistic Approach

Holistic health is more than a collection of practices; it is a philosophy that views health as an intricate tapestry of physical, mental, emotional, and spiritual well-being. This approach recognizes the "holistic triangle" of mind, body, and spirit, emphasizing their interconnectedness. When one aspect falters, the others are affected, much like a symphony where every instrument contributes to the melody. Balance, therefore, is not merely a goal but a way of living, a dynamic state where all parts of ourselves work in harmony to achieve optimal health.

The roots of holistic health run deep, tracing back to ancient practices that have stood the test of time. Ayurveda and Traditional Chinese Medicine (TCM) are two of the oldest systems, each offering a unique perspective on health and healing. According to a study published by the National Center for Biotechnology Information, both Ayurveda and TCM focus on patient-centered health rather than disease, using holistic approaches to treatment. These traditions emphasize the importance of balance, using natural remedies and lifestyle changes to promote health. As modern medicine grapples with the limitations of treating symptoms, there is a resurgence of interest in these ancient systems. People are seeking alternatives that offer a more comprehensive approach to health.

Embracing a holistic lifestyle offers a myriad of benefits. It enhances mental clarity, bringing a sense of peace and focus that many of us crave in a chaotic world. Emotional stability follows, as holistic practices encourage us to process emotions in a healthy way. A strengthened immune system is another benefit, as holistic health promotes practices that support the body's natural defenses. This lifestyle is preventive, reducing the risk of chronic diseases by encouraging habits that support long-term well-being.

However, pursuing holistic health is not without its challenges. Misconceptions abound, with some viewing it as unscientific or mystical. Skepticism can be a formidable barrier, especially for those accustomed to conventional methods. Yet holistic health is grounded in evidence and centuries of practice. The challenge lies in integrating these practices into our modern lives, which are often dictated by schedules and responsibilities. But small, intentional changes can lead to significant transformations.

For those unsure where to begin, understanding the core principles of holistic health is crucial. It involves recognizing the interconnectedness of body, mind, and spirit, and striving for balance in each area. This book offers practical solutions to help you incorporate holistic practices into your daily routine, making it accessible even for the busiest individuals. By the end of this chapter, you will have a deeper understanding of holistic health and be equipped with the tools to begin integrating it into your life.

1.2 The Mind-Body Connection

In recent years, the scientific community has shed light on a fascinating concept: the mind-body connection. This principle suggests that our mental states and physical health are deeply intertwined, each influencing the other in profound ways. At the heart of this relationship lies the nervous system, a complex network that facilitates communication between the brain and the rest of the body. Neuroplasticity, the brain's incredible ability to reorganize itself by forming new neural connections, plays a pivotal role in how we adapt to changes, learn new skills, and recover from injuries. This adaptability allows our mental states to influence physical health and highlights the dynamic nature of human wellness.

One powerful application of the mind-body connection is mindfulness meditation. This practice, which involves focusing attention on the present moment with acceptance and without judgment, has been shown to reduce stress significantly. Research supports the idea that by calming the mind, we can influence physical processes such as lowering blood pressure and reducing the body's response to stress. In practical terms, mindfulness can be as simple as spending a few minutes each day in quiet contemplation, focusing on your breath or the sensations in your body. This practice not only reduces stress but also enhances emotional resilience and mental clarity.

Biofeedback techniques provide another avenue to leverage the mind-body connection for health improvement. By using electronic monitoring devices, individuals can gain awareness of physiological functions such as heart rate or muscle tension, and learn to control them consciously. This technique has shown promise in managing chronic pain, where patients learn to modulate their body's response to stressors, thus reducing discomfort. The ability to consciously influence one's own physiological state underscores the power of the mind-body connection and its potential for improving health outcomes.

The interplay between psychological and physical health is bidirectional. Stress and anxiety, for instance, can manifest as physical ailments like tension headaches or digestive issues. The body's stress response, which originally evolved to protect us from immediate dangers, can become maladaptive when triggered by everyday stressors. Understanding this interaction helps us see how mental health directly impacts physical well-being. It also highlights the importance of addressing both aspects in any treatment plan.

Mental exercises such as visualization can also enhance physical abilities. Athletes often use visualization techniques to improve performance, mentally rehearsing their movements to enhance muscle memory and focus. This cognitive training can lead to real improvements in physical performance, as the brain's motor circuits are activated during mental rehearsal in a way similar to physical practice. Visualization not only boosts confidence but also prepares the body for optimal performance.

The mind-body connection offers a holistic perspective on health, recognizing that our thoughts, emotions, and physical states are interconnected. By engaging in practices that nurture this connection, we can foster overall well-being. Whether through mindfulness meditation, biofeedback, or visualization, these approaches empower individuals to take an active role in their health, bridging the gap between mind and body in a meaningful way.

1.3 Exploring Spiritual Wellness

In the tapestry of holistic health, spiritual wellness is a thread that weaves through every aspect of our lives, offering depth and meaning. It transcends religion, though it may include religious practices for some. Instead, spiritual wellness is about finding purpose and meaning, a quest that guides our actions and infuses our lives with significance. It asks us to look beyond the mundane and explore the values and beliefs that shape our existence. This pursuit of meaning is a deeply personal journey, one that encourages us to reflect on our place in the world and how we connect with others.

Various practices nurture spiritual growth, each offering unique pathways to deepen our understanding and connection to the world around us. Meditation and contemplation are two such practices, allowing us to pause and listen to the innermost whispers of our hearts. In moments of stillness, we can engage with our thoughts and feelings, gaining insight and clarity. Journaling is another powerful tool for self-reflection, providing a private space to explore our emotions and experiences. By writing down our thoughts, we can better understand our journey and learn from it. Community involvement and volunteerism also play pivotal roles in spiritual growth. By engaging with others and contributing to the greater good, we cultivate empathy and compassion, enriching our spiritual lives. These practices remind us of our interconnectedness and the impact we can have on the world.

Spiritual wellness profoundly influences our daily lives, shaping how we interact with others and perceive the world. It fosters enhanced empathy, allowing us to understand and share the feelings of others more deeply. This empathy naturally leads to greater compassion, encouraging us to act with kindness and understanding. As our spiritual wellness grows, so does our ability to form meaningful relationships and create positive change. It enables us to navigate life's challenges with grace, providing a sense of peace and resilience. By integrating spiritual wellness into our lives, we can find balance and harmony, even amidst chaos.

Despite its benefits, achieving spiritual wellness can be challenging. Cynicism and skepticism often obscure the path, fueled by a world that prioritizes tangible results over inner growth. Many individuals struggle to find time for spiritual practices in the noise of everyday life. However, these challenges are not insurmountable. By acknowledging our skepticism, we can begin to understand its roots and address it. It is important to approach spiritual wellness with an open mind, recognizing that the journey is personal and unique to each individual. Small steps, such as setting aside a few minutes each day for reflection or engaging in community service, can gradually lead to profound changes.

As we embrace spiritual wellness, we open ourselves to new possibilities and perspectives. It invites us to explore the deeper questions of life, to seek understanding and connection beyond the surface. The path may not always be clear, but it is rich with potential for growth and transformation. By nurturing our spiritual well-being, we align ourselves with a greater purpose, finding harmony within ourselves and the world around us. This exploration of spiritual wellness is an integral part of holistic health, offering a gateway to a more fulfilling and balanced life. It encourages us to be curious, to question, and to discover the beauty and depth of our inner world. As we continue to explore, we realize that true wellness is not just about the body or mind, but about nourishing the spirit as well, creating a life that is both meaningful and enriching.

Chapter 2
Integrating Holistic Practices into Busy Lives

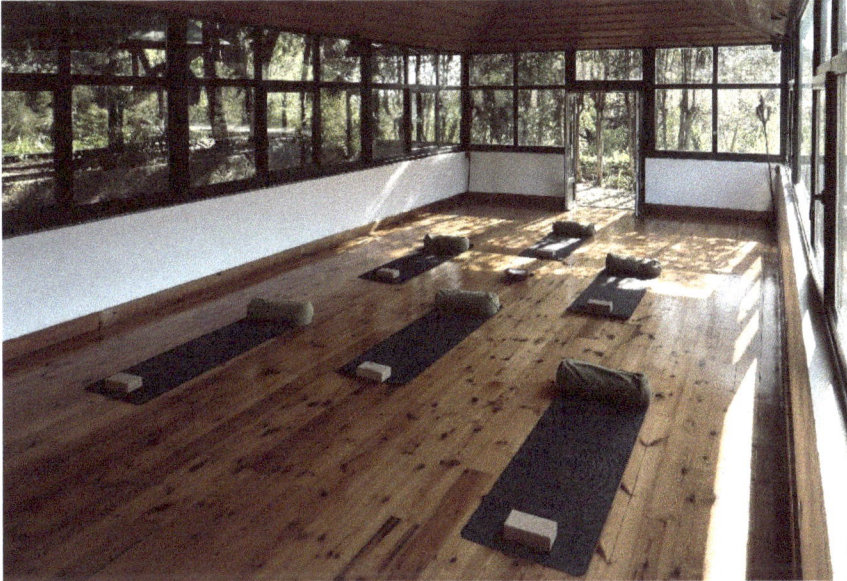

Life can often feel like a whirlwind. The demands of work, family, and personal commitments leave little room for self-care. I recall a particularly hectic week at the hospital, my schedule packed with back-to-back consultations. My stress levels were soaring, and I felt disconnected from myself. It was during one of these frenzied days that I stumbled upon the concept of micro-meditations. Initially skeptical, I was surprised by the profound effect of a simple one-minute pause. This tiny oasis of calm became my refuge, a way to center myself amidst the chaos. I invite you to explore how these brief meditative moments can transform your daily life.

2.1 Micro-Meditations for Stressful Days

Micro-meditations present a revolutionary approach to mindfulness for those who feel they lack time for traditional meditation. These are brief, intentional pauses, lasting just one to five minutes, designed to fit seamlessly into your day. Unlike longer meditation sessions that require dedicated time and space, micro-meditations can be practiced anywhere, from your desk at work to the bus ride home. The essence lies in pausing, breathing, and centering yourself in the present moment. This simple act can activate your body's relaxation response, countering the effects of chronic stress and fostering a sense of calm and clarity.

The techniques involved in micro-meditations are straightforward yet powerful. Begin by closing your eyes, if possible, and taking a deep breath in through your nose, allowing your lungs to fill completely. Hold the breath for a moment before exhaling slowly through your mouth. Focus on the sensation of the breath moving in and out, anchoring your attention in the present. This can be repeated several times, each cycle bringing a deeper sense of peace. For those who find it hard to focus, counting the breaths can help maintain attention. Alternatively, you might try a body scan, briefly checking in with different parts of your body and releasing any tension you notice. These techniques require minimal time and can be practiced discreetly, making them ideal for busy environments.

The benefits of short meditations are both immediate and cumulative. You may notice an instant lift in mood, as the practice shifts your focus away from stressors and into the present. Over time, regular micro-meditations can improve focus and concentration, enhancing your ability to tackle tasks with clarity and precision. This enhanced mindfulness can lead to better decision-making and increased productivity, as your mind becomes more adept at filtering distractions. Moreover, the practice promotes emotional resilience, helping you respond to challenges with a calm and balanced mindset.

Integrating micro-meditations into your daily routine is simpler than you might think. Consider using natural breaks in your day as opportunities to practice. During work, you can take a minute or two to breathe deeply and reset your focus. Commutes provide another perfect chance to engage in micro-meditation; close your eyes and breathe deeply while riding the train or bus. Even mundane tasks like waiting in line or taking a coffee break can become moments of mindfulness. By weaving these practices into your daily rhythm, you create pockets of peace that accumulate to enhance your overall well-being.

Tools and Resources

To support your practice, a variety of digital tools are available. Mobile apps like Headspace and Calm offer a range of guided micro-meditations tailored to fit into busy schedules. These apps provide structured guidance, helping you develop a consistent practice even when time is scarce. They offer reminders and track your progress, encouraging regular engagement. By leveraging these resources, you can make micro-meditations a sustainable part of your lifestyle, ensuring that even amidst the busiest days, you find moments of peace and clarity.

2.2 Quick and Balanced Meal Prep

Eating well doesn't have to be a daunting task, nor should it consume hours of your day. With the right approach, creating quick, balanced meals can become an achievable part of your routine. At the heart of any nutritious meal lies the principle of macronutrient balance. This means ensuring that your meals contain a healthy mix of proteins, carbohydrates, and fats. Proteins help build and repair tissues, carbohydrates provide energy, and fats support cell function. When these macronutrients are in harmony, they fuel your body effectively.

Incorporating seasonal and local produce can further elevate your meals. Seasonal foods are often fresher, more flavorful, and packed with nutrients, while local produce supports sustainability and reduces environmental impact. It is also important to listen to your body's hunger signals and stop eating before you feel completely full. This mindful approach prevents overeating and aids digestion. Consider the timing of your meals as well. Try to avoid heavy, late dinners, which can disrupt sleep. Instead, a lighter evening meal can promote better rest. Additionally, start your day by drinking warm water on an empty stomach. This simple habit aids digestion and hydrates your body after a night of rest.

Efficient meal planning is a game-changer for busy individuals. One effective strategy is batch cooking. By preparing large quantities of food at once, you can save time and effort throughout the week. Cook a big pot of soup, stew, or grains, and store portions in the refrigerator or freezer for later. This method not only saves time but also ensures you have nutritious options readily available. Using versatile ingredients is another smart tactic. Foods like roasted vegetables, quinoa, or grilled chicken can be used in multiple dishes, from salads to wraps. This flexibility simplifies meal prep and keeps your meals interesting. Planning meals in advance reduces the stress of last-minute decisions and helps maintain nutritional quality.

Incorporating time-saving cooking techniques can further streamline your meal prep. One-pot meals and sheet pan dinners are excellent choices. They require minimal cleanup and allow flavors to meld beautifully. Simply toss your ingredients together and let them cook while you attend to other tasks. Kitchen gadgets like slow cookers and pressure cookers are also invaluable. They require minimal supervision and can produce delicious, tender meals. Imagine setting up a slow cooker in the morning and returning home to a ready-to-eat dinner. These tools enable you to prepare healthy meals with ease, even on the busiest days.

Practical meal ideas can make a world of difference in your daily routine. For breakfast, consider overnight oats. Combine oats with your favorite milk, add some fruits and nuts, and let them sit in the fridge overnight. In the morning, you will have a nutritious, ready-to-eat meal. For lunch or dinner, try a stir-fried vegetable dish with tofu and quinoa. It is quick to prepare, packed with protein, and full of flavor. The vegetables offer vitamins and minerals, while the tofu and quinoa provide a plant-based protein source. This type of meal is not only satisfying but also supports holistic health by combining nutritious ingredients in a balanced and delicious way.

2.3 Time-Efficient Exercise Routines

In our fast-paced world, finding time for exercise can seem daunting. Yet, it remains a cornerstone of holistic health, vital for both physical and mental well-being. High-Intensity Interval Training (HIIT) is one solution that offers maximum benefits in minimal time. This form of exercise alternates short bursts of intense activity with periods of rest or low-intensity movement, making it an efficient workout. A typical HIIT session can be as brief as 15 minutes, yet it can boost your metabolism, improve cardiovascular health, and increase muscle strength. Imagine starting with a quick warm-up, followed by a series of exercises like squat jumps, burpees, and high knees, each performed for 30 seconds with short breaks in between. This not only elevates your heart rate but also enhances calorie burn long after the workout is over.

For those pressed for time, incorporating movement into daily activities is a practical way to maintain fitness. Simple desk exercises can break the monotony of long hours at work. Consider shoulder shrugs, seated leg lifts, or even a few minutes of stretching to relieve tension. Walking meetings are another innovative approach, transforming a routine conversation into an opportunity for physical activity. These small changes, though seemingly minor, can accumulate to make a significant impact on your health. They encourage a more active lifestyle without requiring dedicated gym time and can fit seamlessly into your day.

Choosing the right exercise routine involves considering your schedule, preferences, and goals. Home workouts offer flexibility and convenience, allowing you to exercise at your own pace and time. These can range from yoga sessions to bodyweight exercises that require no equipment. On the other hand, gym sessions provide access to a variety of equipment and classes, which can be motivating for some. The key is to find a balance that suits your lifestyle. Yoga, known for its physical and mental benefits, is a versatile option that can be practiced anywhere. Whether you have 10 minutes or an hour, yoga can adapt to your needs, promoting flexibility, strength, and mindfulness.

Staying motivated and tracking your progress are crucial to maintaining a consistent exercise routine. Fitness trackers and apps can be invaluable tools, providing insights into your activity levels, heart rate, and even sleep patterns. They offer a visual representation of your progress, which can be encouraging and help maintain momentum. Setting realistic goals and milestones is equally important. Start small and gradually increase your targets as you build strength and endurance. Celebrate these achievements, no matter how minor they may seem. Remember, progress is personal and varies for everyone. The journey to improved fitness is not a race but a personal commitment to health and well-being.

Incorporating exercise into your life is about finding what works best for you. It is about making small, sustainable changes that align with your goals and lifestyle. By choosing time-efficient methods like HIIT, integrating movement into daily tasks, and selecting exercises that fit your schedule, you can enhance your physical health without sacrificing other aspects of your life. Tracking progress helps you stay motivated and ensures you remain on the path to holistic health. Each step you take, no matter how small, brings you closer to a balanced and fulfilling life.

As we conclude this chapter, remember that integrating these practices into your life is a journey toward balance and well-being. Whether through micro-meditations, balanced meals, or time-efficient exercise, each step contributes to a holistic approach to health. In the next chapter, we will delve into the importance of nutrition and explore how food can be a powerful ally in achieving holistic health.

Chapter 3
Nutrition for Holistic Living

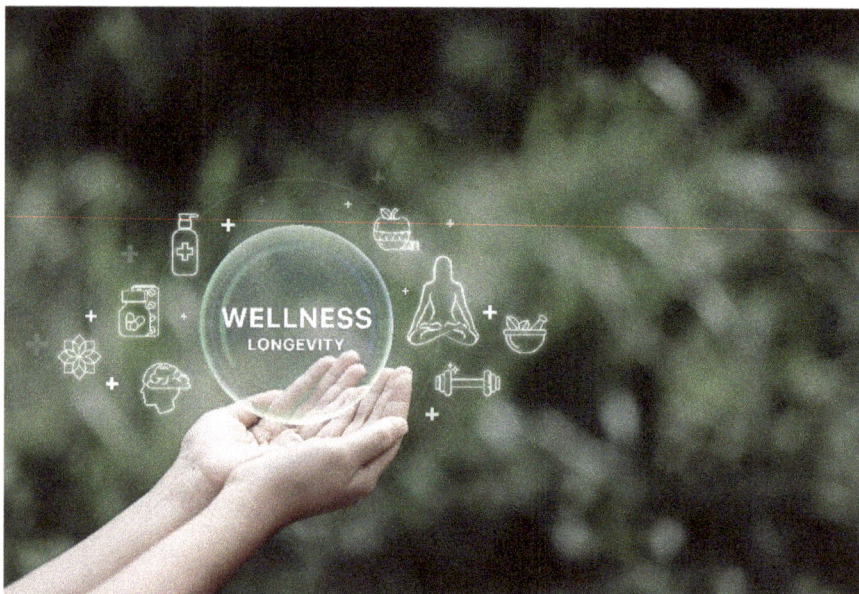

As a medical student, I vividly remember a lecture on nutrition that left me questioning everything I knew about food. The professor spoke of the power of whole foods and their ability to heal and nourish the body in ways that pills and procedures could not. At that moment, I realized the profound impact of what we choose to eat. It wasn't just about satisfying hunger; it was about fueling our entire being. This revelation ignited a passion for holistic nutrition, a journey that has shaped my approach to health and wellness ever since.

3.1 The Power of Whole Foods

Whole foods are the foundation of a holistic approach to nutrition. These are foods that remain close to their natural state, minimally processed, and free from the additives that characterize much of the modern diet. Unlike processed foods, which are often stripped of their nutrients and packed with artificial ingredients, whole foods are rich in essential nutrients that the body needs to thrive. They provide a balanced supply of vitamins, minerals, fiber, and antioxidants, offering a symphony of nourishment that supports overall health. The simplicity of whole foods lies in their authenticity; they are nature's bounty, intended to fuel our bodies and minds.

The nutritional benefits of whole foods are manifold. When you consume whole foods, you are not just filling your stomach; you are enhancing your digestion and gut health. The fiber found in whole grains, fruits, and vegetables aids in digestion, ensuring that nutrients are effectively absorbed while waste is efficiently eliminated. A diet rich in whole foods also lowers the risk of chronic diseases such as heart disease and diabetes. These foods help regulate blood sugar levels, reduce inflammation, and improve cardiovascular health, creating a protective shield against illness. By prioritizing whole foods, you are investing in your long-term well-being, nurturing a body that is resilient and vibrant.

Incorporating whole foods into your diet doesn't have to be complicated. Start by substituting refined grains with their whole-grain counterparts. Swap white rice for brown rice, choose whole wheat bread over white, and explore the versatility of quinoa and oats. These simple changes can significantly increase the nutritional value of your meals. Embrace the abundance of fruits and vegetables, making them the star of each meal. Whether it is a handful of fresh berries with breakfast or a generous serving of leafy greens with dinner, these additions can transform your diet. The key is variety, as each fruit and vegetable offers unique benefits, contributing to a well-rounded intake of nutrients.

Examples of whole foods that deserve a place in your diet are numerous and inviting. Quinoa, with its delightful texture and high protein content, is a versatile grain perfect for salads and side dishes. Brown rice provides a hearty base for stir-fries and bowls, while oats offer a comforting and nutritious start to your day. Leafy greens like spinach and kale are powerhouses of vitamins and minerals, adding color and vitality to your plate. Fresh fruits such as berries and apples are not just delicious but packed with antioxidants, supporting your body's defenses against oxidative stress. By choosing these whole foods, you are aligning with a holistic nutrition philosophy that honors the body's innate wisdom and capacity for health.

A Whole Foods Checklist

To assist you in incorporating whole foods into your daily routine, consider using a checklist. Create a list of whole foods you love and aim to include them in your meals each week. Tick off items as you use them, ensuring variety and balance. This visual aid can serve as a reminder of your commitment to holistic nutrition, keeping you on track as you explore the rich and rewarding world of whole foods.

3.2 Creating Balanced Meal Plans

The key to a balanced meal plan lies in its foundation: the harmonious inclusion of macronutrients such as proteins, carbohydrates, and fats. Each plays a vital role in maintaining health and vitality. Proteins are the building blocks of the body, essential for tissue repair and muscle growth. Carbohydrates, often misunderstood, are the primary energy source, fueling both physical and mental activities. Fats, especially those from healthy sources, support cellular function, hormone production, and nutrient absorption. Achieving the right balance between these macronutrients ensures that your body performs optimally. Portion control is equally important, as it helps maintain a healthy weight and prevents overeating. By listening to your body's hunger signals and adjusting portion sizes, you can enjoy a variety of foods without excess. A well-rounded meal plan also embraces variety, incorporating different flavors, textures, and nutrients, which not only satisfies the palate but also supports diverse nutritional needs.

Building a meal plan that aligns with your nutritional needs and health goals begins with a thoughtful assessment. Consider your dietary requirements, whether you aim to manage weight, increase energy, or address specific health concerns. Reflect on your lifestyle, activity level, and any food preferences or restrictions. Once you have a clear understanding, you can begin planning meals around seasonal produce. Seasonal eating not only enhances the flavor and nutritional value of your meals but also supports local agriculture and sustainability. Incorporating culturally diverse foods can add excitement and novelty to your diet, expanding your culinary horizons and introducing a wealth of nutrients. This approach not only nourishes the body but also enriches the mind.

To illustrate these principles, consider a one-week vegetarian meal plan. For breakfast, you might enjoy a hearty bowl of oatmeal topped with nuts and fresh fruit. Lunch could feature a vibrant quinoa salad with chickpeas, avocado, and a lemon-tahini dressing. Dinner might include a comforting lentil stew served with a side of steamed broccoli. Snacks can be as simple as a handful of almonds or a sliced apple with almond butter. Each meal and snack is thoughtfully composed to deliver balanced nutrients, ensuring sustained energy and satisfaction throughout the day. This structure is merely a blueprint, adaptable to your personal taste and nutritional goals.

Meal plans should never be rigid; they need to adapt to your unique needs. For those managing blood sugar, low-carb options like zucchini noodles with pesto or a grilled chicken salad can be excellent choices. If muscle building is a priority, focus on high-protein meals such as scrambled tofu with spinach and quinoa, or grilled salmon with sweet potato. These adjustments ensure that your meal plan supports your health objectives, providing the right fuel for your body. Flexibility is key, as it allows you to respond to changes in your lifestyle, health status, or preferences.

In crafting your meal plan, remember that it is a tool to support your holistic health journey, not a constraint. It should reflect your individuality and adapt as your needs evolve. Balancing nutrition with enjoyment ensures that your relationship with food remains positive and fulfilling. This approach not only nurtures your body but also fosters a sense of well-being and satisfaction in your daily life.

3.3 Superfoods for Everyday Wellness

Superfoods have garnered attention for their impressive nutritional profiles and health benefits. These nutrient-dense foods are celebrated for their ability to provide a wealth of vitamins, minerals, and antioxidants in every bite. Unlike ordinary foods, superfoods are packed with compounds that actively contribute to health and wellness. Their high nutrient density means that even small portions can deliver substantial health benefits. Antioxidant properties are a standout feature of many superfoods, as they help combat oxidative stress in the body and reduce the risk of chronic diseases. This unique combination of nutrients and antioxidants makes superfoods an invaluable addition to any diet focused on holistic health.

Regular consumption of superfoods offers specific health benefits that are hard to overlook. For one, superfoods are known to boost immune function, thanks to their rich content of vitamins and minerals that support the body's defenses. This makes them an excellent choice for maintaining health, especially during the colder months when illnesses are more prevalent. Additionally, superfoods play a significant role in supporting cardiovascular health. Foods like dark chocolate and avocados contain healthy fats and antioxidants that promote heart health by improving cholesterol levels and reducing inflammation. Incorporating these foods into your diet can contribute to a healthier heart and reduce the risk of cardiovascular diseases, making them a smart choice for anyone looking to enhance their well-being.

Incorporating superfoods into daily meals can be simple and enjoyable. One of the easiest ways to start is by adding chia seeds to your morning smoothies or yogurt. These tiny seeds are packed with fiber, protein, and omega-3 fatty acids, offering a nutritional boost with minimal effort. Turmeric, a vibrant spice known for its anti-inflammatory properties, can be easily added to soups and stews, infusing dishes with both flavor and health benefits. Snacking on nuts and seeds is another practical way to incorporate superfoods into your diet. Almonds, walnuts, and sunflower seeds are rich in nutrients and make for a convenient, satisfying snack. These small changes can have a big impact, enhancing the nutritional quality of your meals without requiring drastic alterations to your diet.

A variety of popular superfoods stand out for their unique health benefits, making them worthy additions to your dietary repertoire. Blueberries, for instance, are often hailed as brain food, thanks to their high levels of antioxidants that support cognitive health and protect against age-related decline. Avocados, with their creamy texture and healthy fats, provide essential nutrients that support heart health and promote satiety. Dark chocolate, when consumed in moderation, offers antioxidants that benefit heart health by improving blood circulation and reducing inflammation. These superfoods are not only delicious but also versatile, easily incorporated into meals and snacks throughout the day. By focusing on these nutrient-rich options, you can enhance your diet and promote a more balanced approach to nutrition.

As we close this chapter, it is clear that superfoods offer a compelling way to elevate your nutrition and support holistic health. Their nutrient density and health benefits align perfectly with the principles of a balanced, holistic diet. By incorporating these foods into your meals, you can enjoy both their flavors and the wellness they promote. In the next chapter, we will explore the art of mindfulness and meditation, delving into practices that support mental clarity and emotional balance.

Chapter 4
The Art of Mindfulness and Meditation

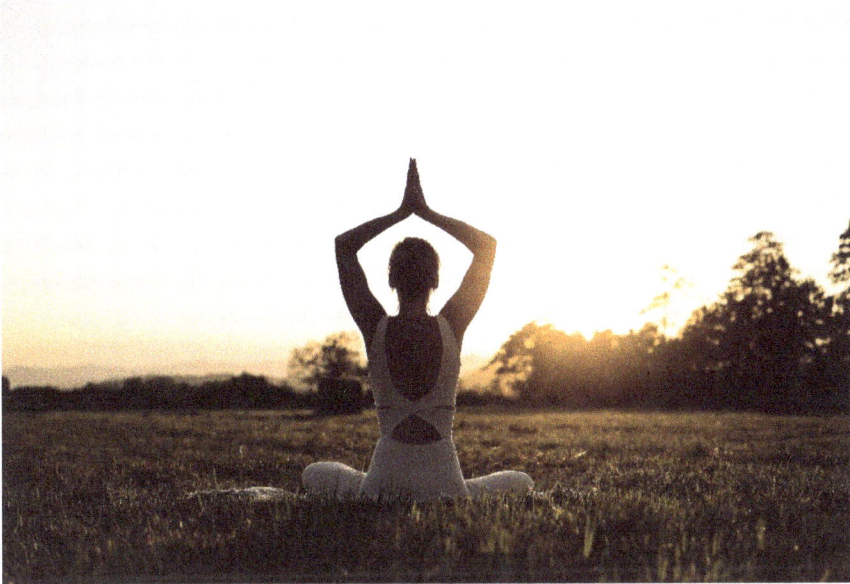

In the bustling corridors of the hospital, amidst the beeping machines and hurried footsteps, I once encountered a patient who changed my perspective on healing. She was an elderly woman, her face lined with years of wisdom and stories untold. Despite her frail condition, she radiated a serene calmness that seemed almost out of place in such a setting. Curiosity piqued, I asked her secret. She smiled gently and spoke of mindfulness, a practice she had embraced for decades. Her words lingered with me, and I found myself compelled to explore this path. It was a journey that led me to a profound understanding of mindfulness and its potential to transform lives.

4.1 Mindfulness for Beginners

Mindfulness is a practice rooted in the simple act of paying attention. It encourages present-moment awareness, a conscious effort to engage fully with the here and now. This involves observing your thoughts, emotions, and sensations without judgment, allowing them to pass through your mind like clouds in the sky. The beauty of mindfulness lies in its accessibility. It requires no special equipment or setting, only the willingness to be present. By focusing on the present, you cultivate a sense of peace and clarity, freeing yourself from the burdens of past regrets and future anxieties.

The benefits of mindfulness are extensive and profound. Regular practice has been shown to reduce stress and anxiety, promoting a sense of calm even amidst life's challenges. This is supported by various studies, including those cited in *Mindfulness Exercises by Jon Kabat-Zinn* (SOURCE 1), which highlight the positive impact of mindfulness on mental well-being. Additionally, mindfulness enhances attention and focus, sharpening your ability to concentrate on tasks and improving productivity. This mental clarity extends beyond the practice itself, influencing all areas of life. As you become more attuned to your thoughts and emotions, you gain a deeper understanding of yourself and your reactions, fostering emotional balance and resilience.

For those new to mindfulness, simple exercises offer a gentle introduction to the practice. Mindful breathing is a foundational technique, inviting you to focus on the rhythm of your breath. Begin by sitting comfortably, closing your eyes, and taking a deep breath in, followed by a slow exhale. Notice the sensation of air entering and leaving your body, anchoring your awareness in the present moment. Another exercise is the body scan meditation, where you systematically focus on different parts of your body, observing any sensations without trying to change them. This practice fosters relaxation and a deeper connection with your body. Additionally, you can infuse mindfulness into everyday activities, such as eating or walking, by paying close attention to the sensations and experiences involved.

Starting a mindfulness practice can present challenges, particularly when faced with distractions and restless thoughts. It is common for the mind to wander, but with patience and persistence, you can gently guide your focus back to the present. Cultivating patience is key, as mindfulness is a skill that develops over time through consistent practice. It is important to approach the practice with a sense of curiosity and openness, allowing yourself to explore without judgment. By embracing the process, you create a space for growth and transformation.

Reflection Exercise

To support your mindfulness practice, consider keeping a reflection journal. Each day, take a few moments to jot down your experiences and observations. What did you notice during your practice? How did it make you feel? This exercise not only reinforces your commitment but also provides insights into your progress and challenges. Over time, this journal becomes a valuable tool for self-discovery and reflection, deepening your understanding of mindfulness and its impact on your life.

4.2 Guided Meditation Techniques

Guided meditation serves as a comforting hand that leads you through the intricacies of your inner landscape. It is particularly helpful for beginners who may find it hard to focus during meditation. Among the many types available, body relaxation meditations are popular for alleviating stress. These sessions gently guide you to release tension from each part of your body, promoting a profound sense of relaxation. As you listen, you may be encouraged to visualize each muscle softening and stress melting away, creating a state of deep calmness. Then there are visualization meditations, which help you picture your goals as if they are already achieved. By vividly imagining the desired outcome, you engage your subconscious mind, aligning your actions and thoughts with your aspirations. This practice is like creating a mental roadmap that gently steers you toward success. Lastly, loving-kindness meditations cultivate empathy and compassion, both for yourself and others. These meditations often involve repeating affirmations of goodwill and kindness, fostering a sense of interconnectedness and warmth. As you extend these positive intentions outward, you nurture a spirit of empathy and acceptance within.

Choosing the right guided meditation is like finding a good book that resonates with where you are in life. Meditation apps offer a treasure trove of options, with diverse categories tailored to specific needs and moods. Apps like Headspace and Calm are renowned for their extensive libraries, offering everything from stress relief to sleep enhancement. They provide structured guidance, making it easier to stay focused and engaged. Online platforms also abound with free guided sessions, allowing you to explore different styles and teachers. Whether you prefer the soothing voice of a seasoned meditation instructor or the simplicity of a nature soundscape, the right guide can make all the difference. It is about finding what speaks to you personally, creating a space where you feel comfortable and supported.

One of the most significant advantages of guided meditation is its ability to provide structure and focus. For those new to meditation, this guidance can serve as an anchor, preventing the mind from wandering. The gentle prompts and visualizations create a framework that fosters deeper relaxation and concentration. As you listen, the guide's voice becomes a soothing presence, helping you navigate through layers of tension and distraction. This can lead to enhanced visualization, where images and sensations become more vivid and impactful. The result is a more immersive experience, where you can explore your inner world with clarity and openness.

Creating your own guided meditation can be a rewarding and empowering experience. Start by identifying your goals or preferences. What do you hope to achieve or feel during your session? Once you have a clear intention, write a script that incorporates calming and positive affirmations. These affirmations should resonate with your desired state, gently guiding you toward it. For example, if relaxation is your goal, your script might include phrases like "I am at peace" or "My body is calm and relaxed." After crafting your script, consider recording it using a soft, soothing voice. Ambient music or natural sounds can enhance the experience, creating an atmosphere conducive to relaxation and reflection. With your personalized guided meditation, you have a tool that speaks directly to your needs, offering comfort and support whenever you seek it. By tailoring the experience to your unique preferences, you cultivate a meditation practice that is both personal and effective.

4.3 Developing a Personal Mindfulness Practice

Creating a personal mindfulness practice begins with establishing a routine that fits seamlessly into your daily life. This doesn't mean you have to set aside hours each day; even a few minutes can make a difference. Start by choosing specific times for your practice, such as morning or evening, when you can dedicate uninterrupted moments to mindfulness. This consistency helps anchor the practice in your daily routine, making it a habit rather than a chore. You might find it helpful to integrate mindfulness into existing routines. For example, take a mindful pause during your morning coffee or practice mindful breathing while commuting. These small changes can transform ordinary moments into opportunities for mindfulness, enriching your day with calm and awareness.

Tracking your progress is a valuable way to maintain motivation and see how far you've come. One effective method is keeping a mindfulness journal. This doesn't have to be a detailed account; even brief reflections on your experiences can be insightful. Write about what you noticed during your practice, how it made you feel, and any challenges you faced. Over time, this journal becomes a personal record of growth, highlighting patterns and improvements that might otherwise go unnoticed. Additionally, using mindfulness apps can aid in tracking sessions and improvements. Many apps offer features that allow you to log your practices, set goals, and receive reminders. Seeing your progress in a tangible way can boost your motivation and commitment.

As your practice evolves, you may wish to explore more advanced mindfulness techniques. Silent retreats offer an immersive experience, allowing you to engage deeply with mindfulness without the distractions of daily life. These retreats provide a structured environment where you can practice intensively, often leading to profound insights and personal growth. Another technique is open-awareness meditation, which involves observing thoughts and sensations without attachment. This practice encourages a state of presence and acceptance, helping you recognize the transient nature of thoughts and emotions. By letting go of judgment, you cultivate a sense of peace and equanimity, deepening your mindfulness practice.

Life is dynamic, and your mindfulness practice should be flexible enough to adapt to changes and challenges. Whether you're navigating a new job, a move, or personal transitions, adjusting your practice to fit your current circumstances is key. This might mean changing the duration or frequency of your sessions or exploring different mindfulness techniques that resonate with your present needs. During times of stress or uncertainty, mindfulness can be a powerful ally. It offers a way to center yourself and find calm amidst chaos, providing clarity and perspective when you need it most. By approaching mindfulness with flexibility and openness, you ensure that it remains a supportive and enriching part of your life.

In developing your mindfulness practice, remember that it is a personal and evolving journey. Tailor it to your lifestyle, track your progress, and be open to exploring new techniques. As you integrate mindfulness into your life, you will find that it not only enhances your well-being but also enriches your connection to the world around you. This journey is uniquely yours, offering endless possibilities for growth and transformation.

As we conclude this chapter, it's clear that mindfulness offers a path to deeper self-awareness and tranquility. By nurturing your practice, you create a life rich with presence and intention. In the next chapter, we'll explore the realm of natural remedies, delving into how herbs and holistic practices can further support your journey to balanced living.

Chapter 5
Natural Remedies and Herbal Medicine

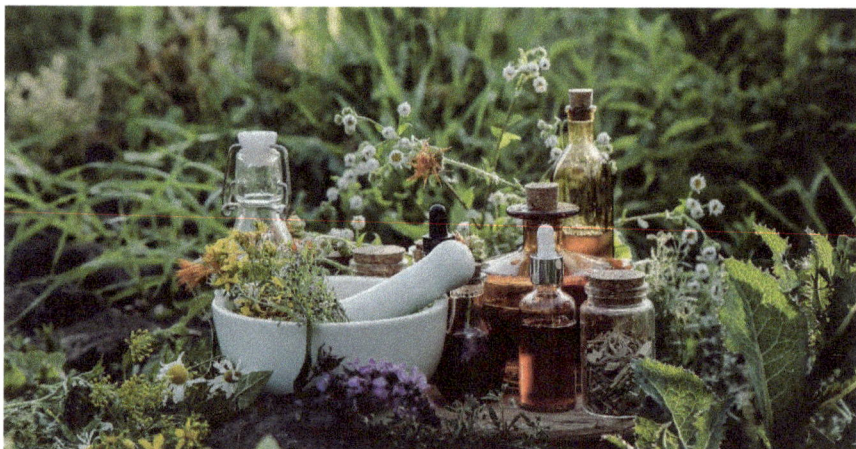

Imagine a lush garden, vibrant with the scents and colors of countless plants, each leaf and petal holding centuries of wisdom within its veins. This garden is not just a sanctuary of nature but a living testament to the ancient art of herbal medicine. My first encounter with herbal remedies took place in a small village clinic, where a local healer brewed a simple tea from leaves she had gathered that morning. The aroma was earthy and comforting, and as I sipped the warm liquid, I felt an inexplicable sense of well-being. This moment unveiled the profound potential of plants, a potential that has been harnessed across cultures and eras to heal and nurture.

Herbal medicine, or phytomedicine, has roots that extend deep into the annals of history. Ancient Egyptian and Chinese civilizations were among the first to document the use of plants for medicinal purposes, creating detailed pharmacopeias that guided their healing practices. Egyptian papyri reveal intricate recipes for treating ailments, while Chinese herbal texts, such as the *Shennong Ben Cao Jing*, delve into the properties of various herbs. This tradition is not limited to these cultures; indigenous peoples worldwide have long relied on the natural world to sustain their health. Their knowledge, passed down through generations, forms the backbone of modern herbal practices. As we continue to explore and validate these ancient remedies, we find that they offer a wealth of benefits that complement contemporary healthcare.

In today's world, herbal practices have found a place in the holistic health paradigm, offering gentle yet effective solutions for common ailments. Herbal teas, cherished for their soothing properties, are a prime example. Chamomile tea can calm the mind and aid digestion, while peppermint tea invigorates and refreshes. These teas harness the natural compounds present in the leaves and flowers, providing a simple way to integrate herbal medicine into daily life. Tinctures, another popular form, offer concentrated herbal benefits. These liquid extracts preserve the active ingredients of plants, making them easily absorbable by the body. A few drops of echinacea tincture can bolster the immune system, while valerian root tincture may promote restful sleep. These practices highlight the versatility and accessibility of herbal medicine, making it an appealing choice for those seeking natural remedies.

The benefits of herbal medicine extend beyond relaxation and digestion. Anti-inflammatory herbs like turmeric and ginger have gained recognition for their ability to reduce pain and swelling. Turmeric, with its active compound curcumin, offers potential relief from arthritis and other inflammatory conditions. Ginger, known for its warming properties, can alleviate nausea and improve circulation. Adaptogenic herbs, such as ashwagandha, help the body adapt to stress, enhancing resilience and energy levels. These herbs support the body's natural ability to maintain balance, offering a holistic approach to wellness. Their applications are numerous, addressing both acute symptoms and promoting long-term health.

To fully benefit from herbal medicine, selecting high-quality herbs is crucial. The market is flooded with products of varying quality, making it essential to choose wisely. Look for organic certifications, which indicate that the herbs have been grown without synthetic pesticides or fertilizers. Understanding labeling can also be helpful; reputable brands often provide information about the herb's origin and processing. Transparency in sourcing and production ensures that the herbs you choose are free from contaminants like heavy metals, which can compromise their efficacy and safety. Proper storage, away from light and moisture, preserves their potency and allows you to enjoy their full therapeutic benefits.

Herbal Medicine Checklist

- **Research Reputable Sources**: Choose brands that provide detailed information about sourcing and production.
- **Check for Certifications**: Look for organic and quality certifications on packaging.
- **Read Labels Carefully**: Ensure transparency in ingredient lists and understand any claims made.
- **Store Properly**: Keep herbs in a cool, dark place to maintain their freshness and potency.

Herbal medicine offers a gateway to nature's pharmacy, providing a path to health that is both ancient and contemporary.

5.2 Essential Oils for Everyday Use

In the realm of holistic health, essential oils serve as a bridge between the aromatic and therapeutic qualities of plants. These oils are not mere fragrances; they are concentrated extracts that capture the essence of the plant's scent and healing properties. The extraction process is an art and science, employing methods like steam distillation and cold pressing. Steam distillation involves passing steam through plant material, which releases the oils. The steam is then cooled, and the oil is separated from the water. Cold pressing, on the other hand, is typically used for citrus oils and involves mechanically pressing the plant material to extract the oil. This method preserves the delicate compounds that give the oils their distinctive properties. It's crucial to differentiate these from fragrance oils, which are synthetically created and lack the therapeutic benefits of essential oils.

Essential oils have found a place in everyday life due to their versatility and beneficial properties. Aromatherapy is one of the most popular applications, harnessing the power of scent to enhance mood and promote relaxation. A few drops of lavender oil in a diffuser can create a calming atmosphere, while citrus oils like bergamot can invigorate and uplift the spirits. Beyond aromatherapy, essential oils are prized for their topical benefits. They can be used in skincare routines to address minor ailments like acne, dry skin, or inflammation. Tea tree oil, known for its antibacterial properties, is often used to treat blemishes, while chamomile oil can soothe irritated skin. These oils can also be added to bathwater, providing a luxurious and therapeutic soak that pampers both body and mind.

Creating your own essential oil blends offers an opportunity to tailor the benefits to your specific needs. For those seeking energy and focus, a blend of peppermint and rosemary can be invigorating, sharpening concentration and boosting mental clarity. Mix a few drops of each oil with a carrier oil like jojoba to create a refreshing roll-on application. On the other hand, those looking for relaxation may find solace in a blend of lavender and chamomile. These calming oils, when combined, can create a soothing bedtime ritual. A few drops in a warm bath or massaged into the temples can ease tension and promote restful sleep. The process of blending oils allows for creativity and personalization, enabling you to craft concoctions that resonate with your senses and support your well-being.

While essential oils offer numerous benefits, they must be used with care. Their potency means that proper dilution is necessary to ensure safety. Always mix essential oils with a carrier oil, such as coconut or almond oil, before applying them to the skin. For adults, a common dilution ratio is 2 to 3 percent, which equates to about 12 to 18 drops of essential oil per ounce of carrier oil. It is important to avoid applying essential oils directly to sensitive areas like the eyes or mucous membranes, as this can cause irritation. Ingestion of essential oils is generally discouraged unless under the guidance of a qualified professional, as it can lead to adverse reactions. Conducting a patch test by applying a diluted oil to a small area of skin can help determine sensitivity or allergies. By adhering to these guidelines, you can safely enjoy the holistic benefits of essential oils and enhance your daily life with their natural wonders.

5.3 Safe Use of Natural Supplements

In the realm of holistic health, natural supplements serve as vital allies, supporting the complex needs of the body and mind. These supplements encompass a broad spectrum, from vitamins and minerals sourced from nature to the beneficial bacteria found in probiotics. Vitamins and minerals play a pivotal role in maintaining bodily functions, enhancing immunity, and preventing deficiencies that could lead to health issues. Vitamin D, for example, is crucial for bone health and immune function, while magnesium supports muscle and nerve function. Probiotics, on the other hand, are live bacteria that nurture gut health, improve digestion, and boost the immune system. They help maintain a balanced microbiome, which is essential for overall health. Incorporating these supplements into your routine can provide the nutrients your body might lack, supporting a holistic approach to well-being.

Determining your supplement needs requires a thoughtful approach. It is essential to consider your lifestyle, dietary habits, and health goals. Consulting healthcare professionals can provide personalized recommendations, ensuring that the supplements you choose align with your specific needs. A nutritionist or doctor can help identify any deficiencies you might have, using tools like blood tests to assess your vitamin and mineral levels. Recognizing signs of nutrient deficiencies, such as fatigue, brittle nails, or frequent illnesses, can also guide your supplement choices. For instance, persistent fatigue might indicate an iron deficiency, while frequent colds could suggest a lack of vitamin C. By understanding your body's needs, you can make informed decisions about which supplements to incorporate into your diet.

Integrating supplements into your diet involves more than just taking a pill. Timing and absorption are critical to maximizing their benefits. Certain vitamins, like A, D, E, and K, are fat-soluble, meaning they are best absorbed when taken with a meal containing healthy fats. Meanwhile, water-soluble vitamins, such as vitamin C and the Bcomplex group, dissolve in water and are best taken on an empty stomach. Pairing supplements with specific meals can enhance their absorption and effectiveness. For instance, take a vitamin D supplement with breakfast that includes eggs or avocado to boost its efficacy. This thoughtful integration not only ensures you receive the full benefits but also fosters a routine that aligns with your dietary habits and lifestyle.

While supplements offer numerous benefits, it is crucial to use them wisely. Moderation is key, as overuse can lead to adverse effects. Excessive intake of certain vitamins and minerals can cause toxicity, leading to symptoms like nausea, fatigue, or even more severe health issues. For example, too much vitamin A can lead to liver damage, while excessive iron can cause digestive problems. Being aware of potential interactions with medications is equally important. Certain supplements, like St. John's Wort, can interfere with prescription drugs, affecting their efficacy or causing unwanted side effects. It's essential to review potential interactions with a healthcare professional, particularly if you are taking medications for chronic conditions. By approaching supplementation with mindfulness and caution, you can safely reap its benefits and enhance your holistic health journey.

As we close this chapter, remember that natural supplements, when used thoughtfully, can be powerful tools in your holistic health toolkit. They offer support where your diet might fall short, complementing your efforts to achieve balance and wellness. The next chapter will explore the role of stress-reduction strategies and delve into practices that promote mental clarity and emotional resilience.

Chapter 6
Stress-Reduction Strategies

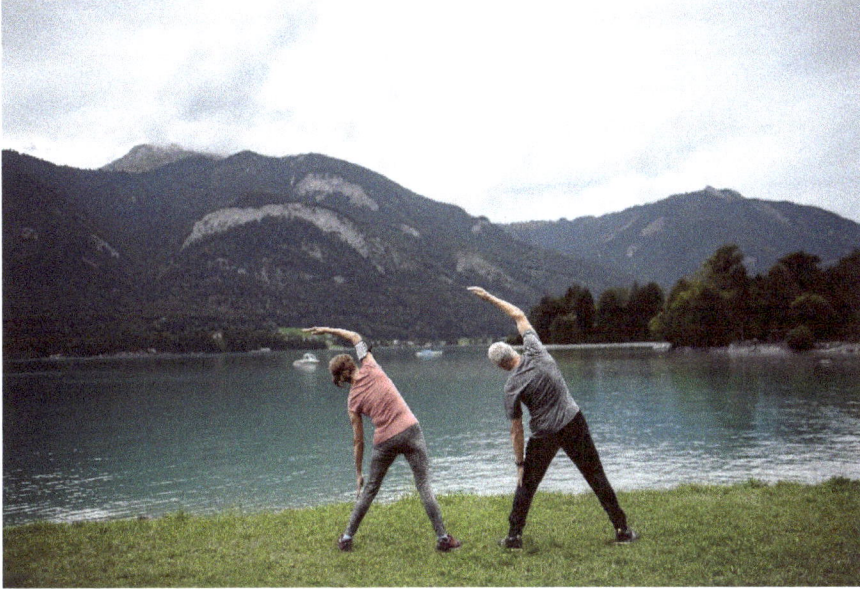

Many years ago, I found myself standing on a sunlit beach, the gentle sound of waves lapping at the shore. The scene was idyllic, yet inside, I was a storm of stress and tension. My mind raced with thoughts of work, deadlines, and the perpetual chaos of life. As I watched the horizon, a group of people began practicing yoga nearby. Their movements were slow and deliberate, each pose flowing seamlessly into the next. Intrigued, I joined them. With each deep breath and stretch, a profound sense of calm washed over me. That day marked the beginning of my exploration into the transformative power of yoga for stress relief, a journey that has not only changed my life but has become a cornerstone of my holistic health practice.

Yoga for Stress Relief

Yoga is a holistic practice that offers both physiological and psychological benefits, making it an effective tool for reducing stress. Its impact begins at the core of our stress response: the autonomic nervous system. By practicing yoga, you can activate the parasympathetic nervous system, often referred to as the "rest and digest" system. This activation encourages relaxation, counteracting the "fight or flight" response that stress triggers. As you move through poses, your body releases tension, and your breathing becomes more regulated, sending signals of safety and calm to your brain.

This physiological shift is complemented by a reduction in cortisol levels, the hormone associated with stress. Lower cortisol levels can lead to improved mood, better immune function, and enhanced overall well-being. On a psychological level, yoga enhances mental focus and emotional stability. The practice encourages mindfulness, drawing your attention away from stressors and fostering a sense of presence and clarity. This mental shift helps build resilience, equipping you to handle life's challenges with greater ease.

The beauty of yoga lies in its diversity, with various styles tailored to meet different needs. For stress relief, certain styles stand out for their soothing and restorative qualities. Hatha yoga, for instance, is characterized by gentle stretching and static poses, making it ideal for those seeking balance and relaxation. It emphasizes proper alignment and breathwork, helping to improve flexibility and strength while calming the mind.

Restorative yoga takes relaxation a step further, using props like bolsters and blankets to support the body in passive poses. This deep rest allows the nervous system to reset, promoting recovery and renewal. Yin yoga, with its focus on long-held poses and deep tissue work, is another excellent choice. It targets connective tissues, releasing tension and fostering a meditative stillness that soothes the mind. Each of these styles offers unique benefits, allowing you to choose the one that aligns best with your needs.

Creating a personal yoga practice begins with setting realistic goals and maintaining consistency. Consider what you hope to achieve, whether it's stress reduction, increased flexibility, or a sense of inner peace. Start with small, attainable goals and gradually build on them as you grow more comfortable with the practice. Consistency is key. Even short sessions practiced regularly can yield significant benefits.

Decide whether you prefer practicing at home or in a studio setting. Home practice offers flexibility and convenience, while studio classes provide guidance and community support. Many online resources and yoga apps can guide you through sessions, offering structured practices that fit into your schedule. Apps like Yoga-X offer free classes tailored to different levels, making it easy to find guidance that suits your experience and goals.

For beginners, certain poses are particularly accessible and effective for stress relief. Child's Pose (Balasana) is a gentle forward fold that promotes relaxation and stretches the back. Start by kneeling on the floor, then sit back on your heels and lean forward, extending your arms in front of you. Rest your forehead on the mat and breathe deeply, allowing tension to melt away.

Legs-Up-the-Wall Pose (Viparita Karani) is another simple yet calming pose. Sit with one hip against a wall, then swing your legs up the wall as you lie back, forming an L-shape. This inversion helps calm the nervous system and encourages circulation.

Cat-Cow Pose (Marjaryasana-Bitilasana) involves alternating between arching and rounding the spine, promoting flexibility and releasing tension. Begin on all fours, aligning your wrists under your shoulders and knees under your hips. Inhale as you arch your back, lifting your head and tailbone. Then exhale as you round your spine, tucking your chin and tailbone.

These poses are not only soothing but also lay the foundation for a mindful yoga practice. Yoga offers a sanctuary of calm amidst the chaos of modern life. By embracing its practices, you can cultivate a sense of balance and serenity, transforming stress into an opportunity for growth and healing. Whether through the gentle stretches of Hatha yoga or the deep relaxation of Restorative yoga, each session becomes a journey inward, fostering resilience and peace.

Tai Chi for Mental Clarity

Tai Chi, often described as "meditation in motion," is a practice that embodies the ancient Chinese philosophy of yin and yang. This concept represents the dual forces that make up the universe, such as light and dark, active and passive, and hot and cold. Tai Chi seeks to harmonize these opposing forces within the body, promoting balance and equilibrium.

The practice originated centuries ago as a martial art, but over time it has evolved into a means of cultivating mental clarity and reducing stress. At the heart of Tai Chi is the principle of flow, where movements are continuous and fluid, much like a gentle stream of water. This focus on harmony in movement helps to quiet the mind, directing attention inward and away from external distractions. As you move through the sequences, you connect with the rhythm of your breath, creating a meditative state that enhances mental clarity and reduces stress.

The benefits of practicing Tai Chi extend beyond physical wellness, offering profound mental and emotional advantages. Regular practice has been shown to improve concentration and memory, making it an excellent choice for those seeking mental clarity. The slow, deliberate movements require focus and precision, engaging both the body and mind in a harmonious dance. This mental engagement helps to sharpen cognitive function, enhancing your ability to concentrate on tasks and retain information.

Tai Chi also fosters enhanced flexibility and balance, crucial components of physical health that often decline with age. The practice gently stretches and strengthens the muscles, improving posture and coordination. Furthermore, Tai Chi is known for its ability to reduce feelings of anxiety and depression. The meditative aspects promote a sense of calm and well-being, while the physical activity releases endorphins that uplift the mood. By incorporating Tai Chi into your routine, you can cultivate a balanced state of mind and body, enhancing overall well-being.

For those new to Tai Chi, starting with basic movements is a practical way to engage with the practice. The Commencing Form is an excellent starting point, designed to ground and focus your energy. Begin by standing with your feet shoulder-width apart, arms relaxed by your sides. Inhale deeply as you slowly raise your arms in front of you, palms facing down, to shoulder height. Exhale as you gently lower your arms back to your sides, visualizing tension melting away. This simple movement sets the tone for your practice, inviting a sense of calm and focus.

Another foundational movement is Grasping the Bird's Tail, which emphasizes balance and flow. From a standing position, shift your weight onto your right foot, turning your torso to the left as you extend your right arm forward in a gentle arc. Your left arm follows, creating a sense of flow and continuity. This movement encourages the mind to focus on balance and coordination, fostering a state of meditative awareness. By practicing these movements regularly, you can build a strong foundation for your Tai Chi practice, enhancing both mental and physical clarity.

Incorporating Tai Chi into your daily life need not be a daunting task. Short morning routines can set a positive tone for the day, awakening the body and mind with gentle movements. Begin each day with a brief session, practicing a few movements to invigorate your body and focus your mind. These morning practices can help you carry a sense of calm and clarity throughout the day, preparing you to face challenges with balance and composure.

Midday practices offer an opportunity to rejuvenate, providing a break from the hustle and bustle of daily life. A few minutes of Tai Chi during lunch can refresh your energy, restore focus, and reduce stress. Evening sessions are equally valuable, offering a way to unwind and prepare for restful sleep. As the day winds down, practicing Tai Chi can help release the tension accumulated throughout the day, promoting relaxation and peace.

By integrating Tai Chi into your routine, you can create a rhythm of balance and clarity that supports your overall well-being. Tai Chi offers a gentle yet powerful approach to enhancing mental clarity and reducing stress. Its principles of balance and harmony, coupled with its physical and mental benefits, make it a valuable addition to any wellness routine. Whether practiced in the morning, midday, or evening, Tai Chi provides a sanctuary of calm and clarity amidst the demands of daily life. As you explore the practice, you will find that each session deepens your connection to yourself, fostering a sense of inner peace and resilience. This exploration of Tai Chi marks a step forward in your journey toward holistic health, paving the way for new discoveries and insights.

Chapter 7
Personalized Holistic Health Plans

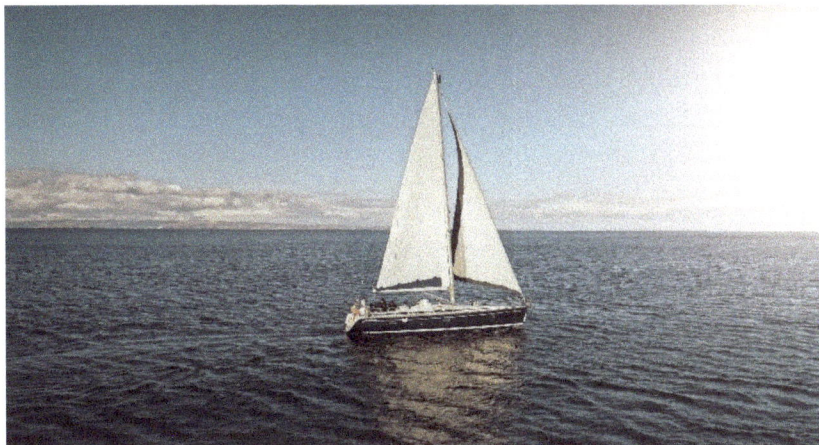

Picture a ship navigating the vast ocean. Without a clear destination, it drifts aimlessly at the mercy of the winds and currents. Much like this ship, our journey toward health requires a defined direction. Setting personal health goals is akin to charting a course, providing the guidance needed to navigate the complexities of a wellness journey. These goals are not arbitrary markers; they are intentional commitments that align with your vision for holistic well-being.

By differentiating between short-term and long-term objectives, you create a roadmap that addresses immediate needs while keeping sight of your broader aspirations. Short-term goals might focus on immediate lifestyle changes, such as incorporating a daily meditation practice, while long-term goals could involve achieving a balanced state of mind, body, and spirit over several months or years. Prioritizing these goals helps you allocate your energy wisely, ensuring that each step builds toward a sustainable and fulfilling lifestyle.

Understanding your current health status is a foundational step in crafting a personalized plan. This involves conducting a thorough self-assessment that includes your physical, mental, and emotional well-being. Reflect on your daily habits, noting patterns that impact your health positively or negatively. Consider using health-tracking tools, such as journals or apps, to gather data on your sleep, exercise, and diet. This information serves as a baseline, helping you identify areas for improvement and recognize existing strengths.

A comprehensive self-assessment offers a clearer picture of your health landscape, enabling you to tailor your plan to your unique needs and circumstances. By acknowledging where you stand, you lay the groundwork for meaningful change and empower yourself to make informed decisions aligned with your holistic goals.

Your lifestyle, shaped by work, family, and social commitments, significantly influences your health needs. Identifying stressors is crucial, as they can create imbalances that affect both physical and mental health. Reflect on your daily routine and consider how factors like job demands or family responsibilities contribute to stress. Recognize how these stressors manifest, whether as tension, fatigue, or emotional strain.

Evaluating the balance between work, leisure, and personal time is equally important. Strive to create a schedule that accommodates relaxation and self-care, fostering a sense of equilibrium amidst life's demands. By understanding the interplay between lifestyle and health, you can make conscious adjustments that support well-being and create a harmonious environment for growth and resilience.

Consulting with health professionals provides valuable insights that enhance your personalized plan. Regular check-ups and health screenings offer a comprehensive view of your physical health, identifying potential risks and areas needing attention. Seek input from specialists like nutritionists or fitness trainers, who can provide tailored guidance aligned with your goals. Their expertise refines your plan and addresses specific challenges.

Additionally, wellness coaches can support your journey by fostering accountability and encouraging sustainable habits. This collaborative approach ensures access to the resources and support necessary to achieve your holistic vision, creating a strong framework that empowers you to thrive.

Reflection Exercise

Take a moment to reflect on your personal health goals. Consider your short-term and long-term objectives, and write them in a dedicated journal. Visualize the steps needed to achieve each goal, breaking them into manageable tasks. This exercise clarifies your intentions and serves as a motivational tool, reminding you of your path. Revisit your goals regularly, adjusting them as your life or priorities change. This practice fosters a dynamic relationship with your wellness journey and empowers ongoing adaptation and growth.

Designing Your Personalized Health Plan

Crafting a personalized health plan is like designing a blueprint for a fulfilling life. It involves creating a balanced framework that addresses every facet of your well-being. This means weaving together physical fitness, nutrition, mental health, and spirituality into a cohesive whole. Imagine each of these as a pillar supporting your overall health: physical fitness energizes the body, nutrition fuels it, mental health fosters resilience, and spirituality provides meaning.

Together, these elements form a holistic approach that nurtures the whole self. Achieving balance requires integrating structured routines with the flexibility needed for spontaneous activities. Life is unpredictable, and your plan should reflect that, offering the stability of routine while allowing space for creativity and adaptation. By embracing both structure and spontaneity, you create a dynamic plan that supports you through every stage of life.

Setting realistic and measurable goals is a crucial step in bringing your health plan to life. The SMART framework—specific, measurable, achievable, relevant, and time-bound—serves as a compass for setting concrete objectives. For example, in the realm of exercise, a SMART goal might be to complete a 20-minute walk five times a week for the next month. This goal is specific in its activity, measurable by frequency and duration, achievable within your lifestyle, relevant to your fitness objectives, and bound by a timeframe.

A nutrition-related SMART goal might involve incorporating two servings of vegetables into each meal for the next six weeks. These goals provide clarity and direction, making it easier to track progress and celebrate achievements. By breaking larger aspirations into smaller, manageable steps, the journey to wellness becomes more attainable and rewarding.

Choosing practices that resonate with your personal preferences is vital for maintaining engagement and enjoyment. Holistic health offers a wide range of practices, each with unique benefits. You might explore tai chi for its meditative movement, yoga for its combination of strength and flexibility, or meditation for cultivating mindfulness. These practices are not one-size-fits-all; they should reflect your interests and health goals.

Beyond traditional methods, include hobbies that promote joy and well-being. Gardening connects you with nature while offering both physical activity and mental relaxation. Artistic pursuits provide creative outlets and space for expression. By selecting activities that align with your passions, you create a plan that feels authentic and fulfilling, encouraging consistency and long-term commitment.

Monitoring progress is essential for keeping your health plan relevant and effective. Keeping a health journal helps document achievements and setbacks, providing insights into what works and what needs adjustment. This practice promotes self-awareness and helps you identify patterns over time. Consider scheduling periodic reviews to reassess your goals and strategies. These reviews act as checkpoints for reflection and realignment.

Life is dynamic, and your health plan should evolve accordingly. Adapt your strategies to reflect changes in your circumstances, interests, or priorities. By regularly evaluating your plan, you ensure it continues to support your needs and align with your evolving wellness vision. This proactive, flexible approach empowers you to take charge of your health and build a life rooted in resilience and well-being.

Adapting Plans for Life Changes

Life, with its unpredictable twists and turns, often demands that we reevaluate and adjust our health plans. Recognizing when these changes are necessary is crucial for maintaining a balanced and effective approach to wellness. Consider life transitions such as career changes or relocation, which can disrupt established routines and introduce new stressors. A promotion might increase your responsibilities, requiring a fresh look at how you manage stress and time. Similarly, relocating to a new city could alter your access to familiar resources, necessitating creativity in finding new ways to stay active and nourished. Family dynamics also play a significant role. The arrival of a new baby, for example, brings joy but also challenges that require adjustments to your schedule and self-care practices. Changes in health status, whether due to aging or new medical diagnoses, further underscore the need for flexibility. A diagnosis might require specific dietary modifications or introduce new physical limitations, prompting a reassessment of your current plan to accommodate these needs.

Incorporating flexibility into your health plan is about preparing for the unexpected and allowing room for spontaneity. Creating backup plans is one strategy to ensure continuity in your health practices during busy or challenging periods. For instance, if you cannot attend your regular gym class, having a set of quick home workouts ready can help keep you on track. Similarly, planning for healthy meals that are easy to prepare ensures that you maintain good nutrition even on hectic days. Flexibility in planning also means allowing for modifications in the intensity or frequency of your activities. If you find that your current exercise routine is overwhelming due to time constraints, consider shorter, more intense workouts or alternate activities that better fit into your schedule. This adaptability ensures that your plan remains practical and sustainable, supporting your overarching health goals without adding unnecessary stress.

A growth mindset is invaluable when navigating changes in your health plan. Viewing challenges as opportunities for growth rather than obstacles fosters resilience and adaptability. Each setback becomes a learning experience, offering insights into what works and what does not. This perspective encourages you to refine your health strategies, making them more robust and effective. For instance, if a particular diet did not yield the expected results, analyze the reasons and adjust your approach, perhaps by consulting a nutritionist or exploring different dietary philosophies. Embracing change with curiosity and openness allows you to evolve alongside your circumstances, ensuring that your health plan remains aligned with your needs and aspirations. This mindset not only enhances your ability to adapt but also cultivates a sense of empowerment, reinforcing your commitment to holistic well-being.

Leveraging support networks amplifies your ability to maintain motivation and accountability during periods of change. Friends, family, and community serve as pillars of support, offering encouragement and shared experiences that enrich your journey. Joining wellness groups or online forums connects you with like-minded individuals who understand the challenges you face. These communities provide a platform for exchanging ideas, sharing successes, and offering mutual encouragement. Engaging with accountability partners can also be beneficial, as they help you stay committed and celebrate your achievements. Regular check-ins with these partners can help you stay focused and provide the encouragement needed to persevere through difficult periods. By tapping into these support systems, you create a network of resources that bolster your resilience and help you navigate life's changes with confidence and optimism.

As you adapt your health plan to life's changes, you create a dynamic framework that supports continuous growth and improvement. This adaptability ensures that your plan remains relevant and aligned with your evolving needs and circumstances. In the next chapter, we will explore the role of the environment in holistic health, examining how your surroundings can influence and support your well-being.

Chapter 8
The Role of Environment in Holistic Health

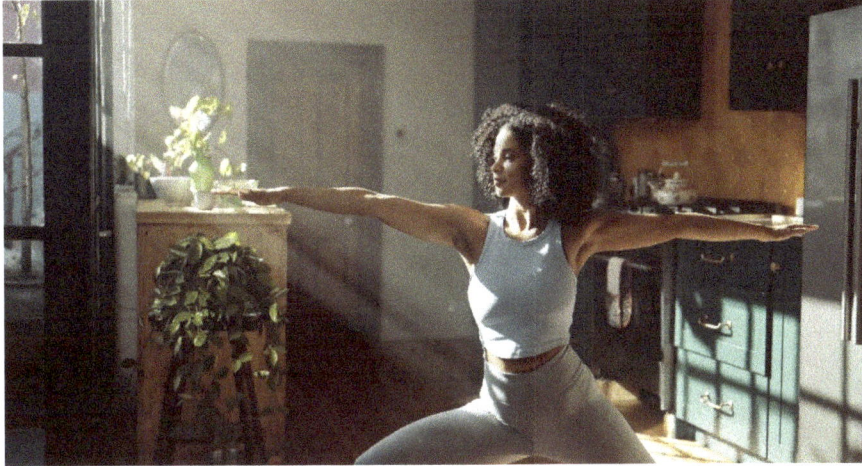

Imagine stepping into a home that feels like a breath of fresh air. The sunlight filters softly through the windows, illuminating a space that feels both serene and invigorating. The air is crisp, carrying the subtle scent of lavender, and the atmosphere exudes a sense of calm. This harmonious environment is not just a matter of aesthetics; it directly influences your well-being. The spaces where you live and work hold the potential to either nurture or deplete your health. Understanding the role of your environment in holistic health empowers you to create spaces that support your journey toward balance and inner peace. As you embark on this exploration, consider how the elements within your home can be transformed to promote optimal health and vitality.

Detoxifying Your Home

Your home should be a sanctuary, yet many common household items release toxins that can undermine your well-being. Volatile Organic Compounds (VOCs), for instance, are prevalent in paints and cleaning products. At room temperature, these compounds vaporize, contributing to indoor air pollution that can irritate the eyes and throat, cause headaches, and exacerbate respiratory problems (SOURCE 1). Synthetic furniture and carpets are also culprits, as they off-gas chemicals that linger in the air, affecting your health long after their newness fades. Additionally, heavy metals like lead can contaminate water sources, posing risks to both your health and the environment. Recognizing these hidden dangers is the first step toward creating a healthier home.

Transitioning to natural cleaning alternatives can significantly reduce your exposure to these harmful substances. Simple ingredients like vinegar and baking soda offer powerful cleaning solutions without the toxic side effects. Vinegar, with its mild acidity, is effective for cutting through grease and grime, while baking soda provides gentle abrasion for scrubbing. Essential oils such as tea tree and lemon add antimicrobial properties, making them excellent choices for disinfection. For specific cleaning needs, consider creating DIY recipes that cater to your home. A mixture of white vinegar and water, for example, makes an excellent glass cleaner, while a paste of baking soda and water can tackle tough stains in the kitchen or bathroom (SOURCE 2). These natural alternatives not only protect your health but also contribute to a more sustainable lifestyle.

Improving indoor air quality is another crucial aspect of detoxifying your home. Investing in air purifiers with HEPA filters can effectively remove airborne particles, including dust, pollen, and pet dander, enhancing your respiratory health. These devices work best in well-ventilated spaces, so consider opening windows regularly to allow fresh air to circulate. Incorporating air-purifying plants, such as spider plants and peace lilies, offers a natural solution to enhancing air quality. According to NASA research, these plants are adept at absorbing pollutants like formaldehyde and benzene, contributing to a fresher and cleaner atmosphere (SOURCE 3). Beyond their purifying capabilities, these plants add a touch of nature and beauty to your home, promoting a sense of tranquility and connection to the natural world.

In our increasingly connected world, electromagnetic fields (EMFs) from electronic devices are an invisible yet pervasive presence in our homes. While the long-term health effects of EMF exposure are still being studied, reducing your exposure can contribute to a more restful and harmonious living environment. Start by limiting the use of wireless devices in bedrooms, where prolonged exposure can disrupt sleep patterns. Opting for wired internet connections over Wi-Fi can also minimize EMF exposure. Consider creating EMF-free zones in your home, particularly in areas designated for relaxation, such as bedrooms or meditation spaces. These zones can serve as sanctuaries, free from the distractions and potential health impacts of electronic devices.

Reflection Exercise

Take a moment to assess your living environment. Reflect on areas where you can reduce toxins and improve air quality. Consider the cleaning products you use, the presence of air-purifying plants, and your exposure to EMFs. Jot down a few changes you can implement over the next month. This exercise not only raises awareness but also empowers you to take actionable steps toward creating a healthier, more balanced home. By aligning your environment with your holistic health goals, you foster a space that nurtures and supports your journey to well-being.

Creating a Zen Living Space

Your home is more than just a shelter; it is a reflection of your inner state and a sanctuary for your soul. Crafting a living space that exudes tranquility and peace can have profound effects on your mental and emotional health. Begin by embracing minimalist decor, which encourages a sense of order and calm. By reducing clutter, you allow the energy in your home to flow freely, creating an environment that feels open and inviting. Think of your space as a blank canvas, where every item has a purpose and place. Incorporate natural materials like wood and stone to add warmth and texture. These elements connect you to the earth, grounding you in moments of chaos. Additionally, a neutral color palette can transform your space into a serene haven. Soft shades of beige, gray, and cream soothe the senses, while subtle accents of color can add interest without overwhelming. Each choice you make in designing your space should support a sense of balance and ease.

Bringing nature indoors is a powerful way to enhance your living environment. The presence of natural elements can positively impact your mood and energy levels, creating a space that nurtures both body and mind. Consider adding indoor water features, like a small fountain, to provide soothing background noise. The gentle sound of flowing water can mask urban noise, promoting relaxation and focus. Strategically arranging plants throughout your home offers both visual appeal and health benefits. They not only beautify your space but also improve air quality, contributing to a healthier living environment. Choose plants that thrive in indoor conditions and require minimal maintenance, allowing you to enjoy their benefits without added stress. Lastly, make the most of natural light, which can elevate your mood and increase energy levels. Position your furniture to maximize exposure to sunlight, and use sheer curtains to diffuse light and create a soft, inviting glow. These elements of nature infuse your home with vitality, fostering a sense of well-being and connection.

To fully embrace holistic living, consider dedicating specific areas of your home to wellness activities. Creating functional spaces for these practices encourages regular engagement and supports a balanced lifestyle. Design a meditation corner with comfortable cushions and soothing elements like incense or a small altar. This space serves as a reminder to pause and reflect, offering a sanctuary for introspection and mindfulness. For those who practice yoga, set up a dedicated area with a mat and essential props, like blocks and straps, to facilitate your practice. This space should be free of distractions, allowing you to focus fully on your movements and breath. A quiet reading nook can also provide a retreat for relaxation and mental rejuvenation. With a cozy chair, good lighting, and a selection of inspiring books, this nook becomes a haven for reflection and personal growth. Each of these spaces should be tailored to your preferences, creating a personalized environment that supports your holistic health journey.

Incorporating Feng Shui principles into your home design can further enhance the harmony and flow of energy. This ancient Chinese practice focuses on creating balance and optimizing the flow of chi, or life energy, throughout your space. Begin by arranging furniture to facilitate smooth movement and energy flow. Avoid blocking pathways or creating obstacles, which can disrupt the natural flow of chi. Mirrors can be strategically placed to expand space and reflect positive energy, brightening dark corners and enhancing the overall atmosphere. When selecting decor, choose items that resonate with your intentions and goals. Each piece should contribute to the harmony and balance of your environment, fostering a sense of peace and well-being. By aligning your space with Feng Shui principles, you create a harmonious environment that supports your holistic lifestyle, enhancing both your home and your inner world.

Creating a Zen living space is about more than aesthetics; it is about nurturing an environment that supports your holistic health and well-being. By embracing minimalist design, incorporating nature, and dedicating spaces for wellness activities, you foster an atmosphere of tranquility and balance. As you continue to explore holistic living, consider how your environment can serve as a foundation for growth and transformation. The next chapter will delve into the importance of holistic health for aging, offering insights and strategies for maintaining vitality and well-being as you navigate life's stages.

Chapter 9
Holistic Health for Aging

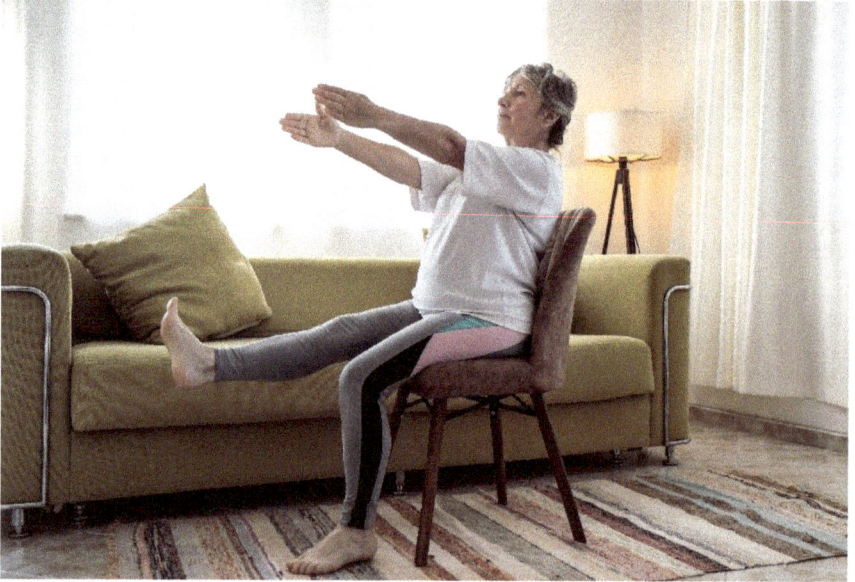

Growing older is a journey marked by wisdom and experience, but it also brings new physical challenges. I remember a patient, Mr. Thompson, who once came to me with a simple wish: to dance at his granddaughter's wedding. At the time, he struggled with mobility, and the idea of dancing seemed distant. Yet, through dedicated practice and the right exercises, he not only danced but did so with a grace that belied his age. His story underscores the power of staying mobile as we age, a crucial factor in maintaining independence and a high quality of life.

9.1 Mobility Exercises for Aging Gracefully

As we age, maintaining mobility becomes more than just a convenience; it is a cornerstone of independence. The ability to move comfortably and confidently can greatly affect your quality of life. Mobility allows you to engage in daily activities, from getting out of bed to exploring the outdoors, without relying on others. It reduces the risk of falls and injuries, which are common concerns that often mark the difference between living independently and requiring assistance. These falls can lead to serious injuries and may be debilitating. Therefore, focusing on mobility can help you stay active and engaged with the world around you, preserving your autonomy and enhancing your enjoyment of life.

For older adults, specific exercise regimens can vastly improve mobility and flexibility. Low-impact exercises, such as swimming and cycling, offer a gentle yet effective means of strengthening muscles and improving cardiovascular health. These activities are easy on the joints, making them ideal for those with arthritis or other joint concerns. They are also enjoyable and often allow for social interaction and a sense of community. Chair yoga provides another excellent option, offering gentle stretching that can improve flexibility without the need for standing poses. It is accessible and can be done at home, making it a convenient option for those who might not be comfortable in a traditional yoga class. Furthermore, Tai Chi is renowned for its benefits in enhancing balance and coordination. Its slow, deliberate movements not only improve physical strength but also promote mental focus and relaxation, offering a holistic approach to health.

Strength training is often overlooked but is essential for maintaining muscle mass and bone density as you age. Simple resistance band exercises are effective and can be done at home with minimal equipment. These bands provide variable resistance, allowing you to tailor the intensity to your ability. Bodyweight exercises, such as wall push-ups, are also beneficial. They require no special equipment and can be easily modified to suit individual needs. These exercises help maintain strength and function, which are crucial for carrying out everyday tasks and preventing frailty. They also contribute to better posture and balance, reducing the risk of falls.

When it comes to exercise, one size does not fit all. It is important to adapt exercises to meet your unique needs and abilities. Using adaptive equipment, like stability balls, can enhance your workout by providing support and increasing the challenge. Modifying exercises to prevent joint strain is equally important. This might mean adjusting the range of motion or using support during certain movements. The key is to listen to your body and work within your comfort zone, gradually building strength and flexibility. By tailoring your exercise routine to your personal needs, you can enjoy the benefits of physical activity without the risk of injury.

Reflection Exercise: Craft Your Mobility Plan

Take a moment to assess your current mobility. Reflect on areas where you feel strong and those where you might need improvement. Consider your daily activities and any challenges you face. Use this insight to craft a personalized mobility plan, incorporating exercises that address your specific needs and goals. Document your plan and set small, achievable milestones. This reflection not only empowers you to take charge of your mobility but also provides a clear path forward in your journey to aging gracefully.

9.2 Cognitive Health in Later Years

Aging gracefully involves more than physical well-being; it encompasses maintaining a sharp and active mind. As we age, cognitive changes are inevitable, but understanding them can help us address them proactively. One common change is age-related memory loss, which often manifests as minor forgetfulness, like misplacing keys or struggling to recall names. While these lapses can be frustrating, they are a normal part of aging. However, lifestyle factors also play a significant role in cognitive health. Stress, poor diet, and lack of mental stimulation can exacerbate cognitive decline. By recognizing these contributing elements, we can take steps to mitigate their impact and support brain health as we age.

Enhancing cognitive function in later years requires engaging the brain in new and stimulating ways. Mentally stimulating activities, such as puzzles, crosswords, and reading, are excellent tools for keeping the mind active. These activities challenge the brain, improving memory and cognitive flexibility. Reading, in particular, exposes the mind to new ideas and vocabulary, fostering continued learning and development. Additionally, learning new skills or languages can provide a significant cognitive boost. When you take up a new hobby or language, the brain forms new neural connections, enhancing its capacity to learn and adapt. This mental workout keeps the brain agile and may delay the onset of cognitive decline.

Social engagement is another crucial element in maintaining cognitive vitality. Interacting with others provides mental stimulation and emotional support, both essential for a healthy brain. Joining community groups or clubs offers opportunities to meet new people and engage in meaningful conversations. These interactions can lead to new friendships and shared experiences, enriching your social life and mental health. Volunteering is also an excellent way to stay socially connected. By contributing to a cause you care about, you gain a sense of purpose and fulfillment, which can positively impact cognitive function. These social connections help reduce feelings of isolation and loneliness, common issues among older adults that can negatively affect cognitive health.

Nutritional support plays a vital role in supporting cognitive function. Certain foods and nutrients are particularly beneficial for brain health. Omega-3 fatty acids, found in fish like salmon and plant sources such as flaxseeds, are known for their anti-inflammatory properties and their ability to support brain health. These healthy fats are essential for maintaining the structure and function of brain cells. Antioxidant-rich foods, like berries and dark chocolate, also provide cognitive benefits. Antioxidants help combat oxidative stress, a factor that can contribute to cognitive decline. Incorporating these foods into your diet can help protect the brain and support mental clarity. A balanced diet rich in these nutrients can contribute significantly to maintaining cognitive health as you age.

Engaging in activities that promote cognitive health is as important as maintaining physical fitness. The brain, like any muscle, requires regular exercise to stay strong and functional. By embracing mentally stimulating activities, fostering social connections, and prioritizing nutrition, you can support your cognitive health and enjoy a vibrant, fulfilling life in your later years.

9.3 Nutrition for Longevity

As we age, our bodies undergo changes that alter nutritional needs, making it crucial to adapt dietary habits to maintain health and vitality. One significant adjustment is the increased need for calcium and vitamin D. These nutrients are vital for bone health, helping to prevent osteoporosis and fractures. As bones naturally lose density over time, ensuring adequate intake becomes paramount. Foods such as dairy products, leafy greens, and fortified cereals can provide calcium, while vitamin D can be obtained from sunlight exposure and foods like fatty fish and fortified milk. The synergy between these nutrients is essential for keeping bones strong and reducing the risk of injury.

Digestive health also becomes more important with age, and fiber plays a pivotal role in maintaining it. Fiber aids in digestion by promoting regular bowel movements and preventing constipation, a common issue among older adults. Incorporating a variety of fiber-rich foods, such as whole grains, fruits, and vegetables, can support a healthy digestive system. These foods not only enhance digestion but also help control blood sugar levels and maintain a healthy weight. By focusing on fiber, you support your digestive tract and contribute to overall well-being.

Superfoods offer a powerful means to support longevity and overall health as we age. Leafy greens like kale and spinach are packed with calcium, vitamin K, and antioxidants, all of which contribute to bone health and help reduce inflammation. Including these greens in your diet can help protect against age-related decline and keep your bones strong. Nuts and seeds, rich in healthy fats, fiber, and protein, support heart health. They provide essential nutrients that help lower cholesterol levels and reduce the risk of cardiovascular disease. Whether sprinkled on salads or enjoyed as a snack, these superfoods can play a significant role in maintaining heart health and promoting longevity.

Hydration is another critical aspect of aging well. As we grow older, our sense of thirst diminishes, increasing the risk of dehydration, which can lead to fatigue, confusion, and more severe health issues. It's essential to encourage regular fluid intake throughout the day. Water should be the primary drink, but herbal teas, milk, and water-rich fruits and vegetables like cucumbers and oranges can also contribute to hydration. Recognizing signs of dehydration, such as dry mouth, dizziness, or dark urine, is crucial for timely intervention. Keeping a water bottle nearby and setting reminders can help maintain adequate fluid intake, ensuring your body functions optimally.

Creating balanced and nutritious meal plans tailored to aging needs is key to supporting longevity. Start by incorporating a variety of food groups to ensure comprehensive nutrition. Include lean proteins, whole grains, fruits, vegetables, and healthy fats in each meal. Portion control is important for maintaining a healthy weight and preventing overeating. Use smaller plates or bowls to help manage portions and avoid the temptation to eat more than necessary. Meal examples might include a breakfast of oatmeal topped with berries and nuts, a lunch of grilled chicken salad with mixed greens, and a dinner of baked salmon with quinoa and steamed vegetables. These meals are not only nutritious but also satisfying and flavorful, making healthy eating enjoyable and sustainable.

By focusing on these nutritional strategies, you can support your body's changing needs and promote longevity. Emphasizing calcium, vitamin D, and fiber, along with incorporating superfoods and staying hydrated, lays a strong foundation for health in later years. As you continue exploring holistic health, remember that nutrition is a powerful tool for maintaining vitality and enhancing your quality of life.

Chapter 10
Emotional and Mental Wellness

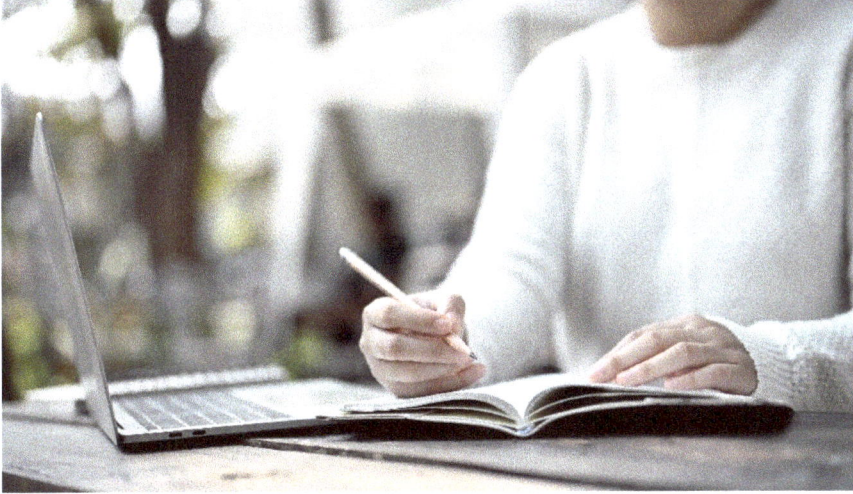

One evening, after a particularly long day filled with patient consultations and endless paperwork, I sat at my desk, feeling a whirlwind of emotions. I found myself reaching for a journal I had not touched in years. As I began to write, pouring my thoughts onto the pages, I experienced a profound sense of relief. It was as if the act of writing allowed me to untangle the knots in my mind, bringing clarity and calm. This personal revelation deepened my appreciation for journaling as a tool for emotional clarity and stress reduction.

10.1 Journaling for Emotional Clarity

Journaling serves as a powerful method for processing emotions, offering a safe space to express feelings freely. When you write, you create a private dialogue with yourself, unencumbered by judgment or expectation. This freedom to express can be cathartic, helping you release pent-up emotions and gain a deeper understanding of your inner world. Moreover, journaling aids in recognizing patterns and identifying triggers that may influence your emotional state. As you review your entries over time, you may discover recurring themes or situations that evoke strong emotions, enabling you to address them more effectively.

Additionally, journaling enhances problem-solving skills and creativity. By exploring different perspectives on paper, solutions to challenges often emerge, as the act of writing stimulates the brain's creative processes. According to a study cited by WebMD, the benefits of journaling extend to mental health, reducing anxiety and promoting well-being by allowing individuals to break cycles of brooding and gain awareness of difficult situations.

Different journaling techniques cater to diverse emotional needs, providing flexibility in how you choose to engage with your thoughts. Stream-of-consciousness writing is one such method, allowing you to write continuously without censorship and offering an outlet for emotional release. This free-flowing style can be liberating, as it encourages you to explore your thoughts and feelings without inhibition. Gratitude journaling, on the other hand, shifts your focus to positive aspects of life, fostering a sense of appreciation and contentment. By regularly noting things you are grateful for, you cultivate a more positive outlook, which can enhance emotional resilience.

Reflective journaling involves revisiting past experiences and processing them through writing to gain insights and understanding. This practice can be particularly beneficial for those seeking to learn from their past and make informed decisions for the future. Each technique offers unique benefits, allowing you to tailor your journaling practice to your personal needs and preferences.

Incorporating journaling into your daily life need not be daunting, even amidst a busy schedule. Begin by setting aside a specific time each day for journaling, creating a routine that becomes a natural part of your day. Whether it's a quiet moment in the morning or a reflective pause before bed, consistency is key. To stimulate writing when you feel stuck, consider using prompts. These can be simple questions or statements that encourage introspection and exploration of specific themes. For instance, prompts like "What am I feeling today?" or "What am I grateful for?" can jumpstart your writing process and guide your thoughts in a meaningful direction. By establishing a regular practice, you create a space for self-reflection and growth, enriching your emotional well-being.

Common barriers to journaling, such as self-criticism and perfectionism, can inhibit the flow of writing. It's important to remember that journaling is a personal endeavor, free from the constraints of grammar or structure. Allow yourself the freedom to write imperfectly, focusing on expression rather than form. Combat self-criticism by approaching your writing with curiosity and acceptance, viewing each entry as a step toward self-discovery. Finding motivation and consistency can also be challenging, especially during busy periods. To overcome this, remind yourself of the benefits journaling brings, using your own experiences as evidence of its value. Some find it helpful to set small, achievable goals, such as writing for just a few minutes each day, gradually building a habit that fits seamlessly into their routine. Adopting this mindset can transform journaling from a task into a rewarding practice that supports emotional clarity and growth.

Reflection Exercise

Take a moment to reflect on your current emotional state. Consider what themes or emotions you would like to explore in your journal. Set a timer for five minutes and write continuously, allowing your thoughts to flow without judgment. Afterward, review what you have written, noting any patterns or insights that emerge. Use this exercise as a foundation to cultivate a regular journaling practice, nurturing your emotional wellness.

10.2 Building Emotional Resilience

Emotional resilience is a remarkable trait, a kind of inner fortitude that allows you to bounce back from life's inevitable setbacks and adversities. It is not about avoiding difficulties but about how you navigate through them. Picture resilience as a tree bending in the face of strong winds without breaking. This flexibility and strength are crucial for maintaining a positive outlook even when circumstances are less than ideal. Emotional resilience enables you to adapt, learn, and grow from challenges rather than being overwhelmed by them. It is the capacity to absorb life's blows and still have the energy and optimism to move forward. In a world where change is constant, resilience becomes your ally and a steady foundation upon which you can rely.

Strengthening emotional resilience is a process that involves both mindset and practice. One effective strategy is to develop a growth mindset, a concept that involves viewing challenges as opportunities for learning rather than insurmountable obstacles. Embracing this mindset encourages you to see failures as stepping stones to success, fostering a willingness to take risks and explore new possibilities.

Coupled with this is the practice of self-compassion and kindness, which involves treating yourself with the same understanding and care that you would offer a friend. When setbacks occur, acknowledge your feelings without self-criticism, and remind yourself that mistakes are part of the human experience. This nurturing attitude not only bolsters resilience but also enhances overall well-being, creating a supportive internal environment where growth and healing can flourish.

A strong support system is another cornerstone of resilience. The people around you, friends, family, and colleagues, play a significant role in your ability to cope with life's challenges. Building and maintaining healthy relationships provides a safety net, offering emotional and practical support when you need it most. These connections create a sense of belonging and community, reminding you that you are not alone. Moreover, seeking support from loved ones or joining support groups can provide invaluable perspectives and encouragement. According to research, social support can enhance resilience by influencing various physiological systems in the body, reducing stress and promoting mental health. This interconnectedness offers strength in numbers, allowing you to draw upon the collective wisdom and experience of those who care about you.

Coping Mechanisms

Coping mechanisms are the tools you use to manage stress and adversity, helping you maintain balance and perspective. Mindfulness meditation is a powerful technique for staying present during tough times. By focusing on the present moment, you can reduce the influence of stressors and cultivate a sense of calm and clarity. This practice involves observing your thoughts and feelings without judgment, allowing you to respond to challenges with greater equanimity. Creative outlets such as art or music also provide effective ways to express emotions and release tension. Engaging in these activities taps into your innate creativity, allowing you to explore and process your feelings in a non-verbal way. Whether it's painting a canvas or playing an instrument, these outlets offer a sanctuary for emotional expression, fostering resilience by providing a means to channel and transform stress into something beautiful and meaningful.

By weaving these strategies into the fabric of your daily life, you can build a robust foundation of emotional resilience. It's about embracing life's challenges with an open heart and a positive mindset, fortified by the support of those around you. As you cultivate resilience, you find yourself better equipped to navigate the ebbs and flows of life, emerging from each experience stronger and wiser.

10.3 Techniques for Anxiety Management

Understanding the origins of anxiety is the first step in managing it effectively. Anxiety often arises from a combination of environmental factors and personal stressors, each contributing to a heightened sense of unease. Imagine walking into a cluttered room filled with noise and chaos. Such an environment can easily trigger feelings of anxiety, as the brain struggles to process the overwhelming stimuli. Similarly, personal stressors, like looming work deadlines or the prospect of a social event, can ignite anxiety. These stressors tap into the mind's fear of the unknown or the pressure to perform, causing a cascade of anxious thoughts. Recognizing these triggers is crucial, as it allows you to take preventive measures, helping you maintain a sense of calm in situations that might otherwise provoke anxiety.

Once you've identified your triggers, it's essential to have tools at your disposal to alleviate anxiety quickly. Breathing exercises offer a simple yet powerful way to calm the nervous system and bring the mind back to the present. Diaphragmatic breathing, also known as belly breathing, encourages deep breaths that engage the diaphragm. This technique can soothe the body by activating the parasympathetic nervous system, which promotes relaxation. To practice, place one hand on your chest and the other on your abdomen. Inhale deeply through your nose, allowing your abdomen to rise while your chest remains still. Exhale slowly through your mouth, feeling your abdomen fall. Repeat this cycle a few times, focusing on the rhythm of your breath. Another effective technique is box breathing, which involves inhaling, holding, exhaling, and pausing for equal counts. Picture a box, and as you breathe, trace its sides with your mind: inhale for four counts, hold for four, exhale for four, and pause for four. This structured breathing pattern can ground you and enhance focus, providing a sense of stability amidst chaos.

Cognitive behavioral strategies offer another layer of support in managing anxious thoughts. These techniques involve challenging and reframing negative thought patterns, which can perpetuate anxiety if left unchecked.

Start by identifying a negative thought, such as "I'll never meet this deadline." Examine the evidence for and against this belief, questioning its validity. Often, you'll find that such thoughts are exaggerated or unfounded. Replace them with more balanced affirmations, like "I can manage my time effectively to meet this deadline." This cognitive restructuring not only alleviates anxiety but also reinforces positive thinking. Additionally, using affirmations can be a powerful tool in this process. Create a list of positive statements that resonate with you, and repeat them daily. Over time, these affirmations can reshape your mindset, fostering resilience and confidence in the face of anxiety.

For long-term anxiety management, lifestyle changes play a pivotal role. Incorporating regular physical activity into your routine is a proven method to reduce anxiety levels. Exercise releases endorphins, the body's natural mood elevators, which can counteract anxiety and promote a sense of well-being. Whether it's a brisk walk, a yoga session, or a workout at the gym, find an activity you enjoy and make it a regular part of your life. Alongside exercise, establishing a consistent sleep routine is vital. Quality sleep is essential for mental health, as it allows the brain to process emotions and rejuvenate. Aim for 7-9 hours of restful sleep each night, creating a bedtime routine that encourages relaxation. Limit screen time before bed, and create a calm sleep environment to enhance your rest. Additionally, be mindful of your intake of caffeine and alcohol. Both substances can exacerbate anxiety, disrupting sleep and increasing nervousness. By reducing consumption, you create a more stable internal environment, supporting long-term anxiety reduction.

This chapter explored practical approaches to managing anxiety, from identifying triggers to employing breathing techniques and cognitive strategies. As you incorporate these methods into your daily routine, you empower yourself to navigate anxiety with greater ease and resilience. These tools not only provide immediate relief but also contribute to a more balanced and fulfilling life. As we transition to the next chapter, we continue to build on these concepts, exploring further how holistic practices can support mental and emotional health.

Chapter 11
Integrative Medicine Insights

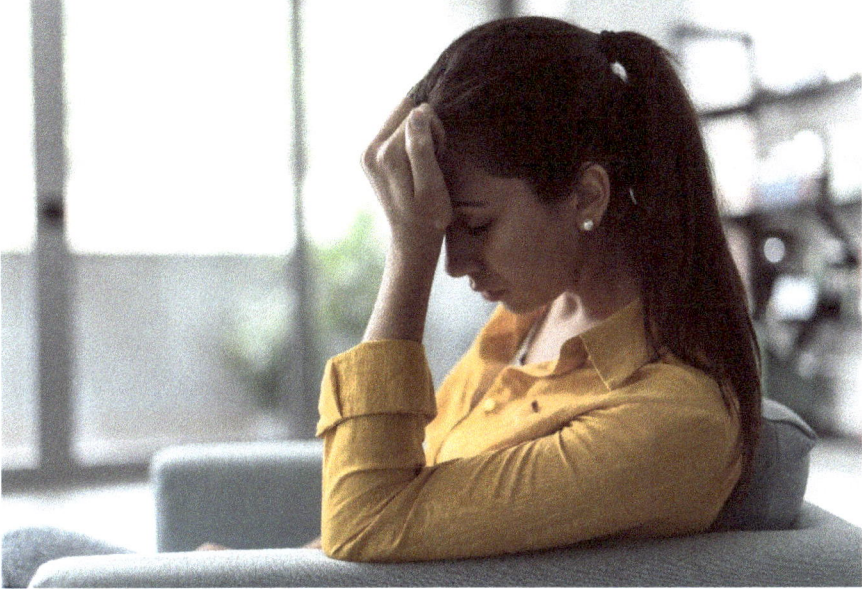

As a young practitioner, I once encountered a patient whose symptoms seemed to defy conventional treatment. Despite numerous tests and medications, her condition persisted. Frustrated, she asked if there was anything else we could try. This moment was pivotal for me, sparking a curiosity that led me into the realm of integrative medicine. This approach combines traditional medical treatments with complementary practices, aiming to treat the whole person, body, mind, and spirit. Integrative medicine doesn't replace conventional care but enhances it, offering a more comprehensive path to wellness. It's about weaving together the best of both worlds, creating a tapestry of care that addresses every facet of health.

11.1 Collaborating with Healthcare Providers

Open communication with your healthcare providers is paramount when incorporating holistic practices into your health regimen. This dialogue ensures that all aspects of your treatment are aligned, maximizing the benefits while minimizing risks. When you visit your doctor, it's crucial to share a complete health history. This includes any holistic practices you are currently following, such as yoga, meditation, or herbal supplements. Being transparent about these practices helps your doctor understand the full picture of your health and avoids potential interactions with prescribed treatments. For instance, certain herbs might affect how medications work in your body. By discussing these factors openly, you and your healthcare provider can make informed decisions that support your overall well-being.

Building a collaborative relationship with your healthcare professionals requires a proactive approach. Before appointments, take the time to prepare questions and concerns. Write them down to ensure you address everything during your visit. This preparation helps you make the most of your time with your doctor and ensures you leave with a clear understanding of your health plan. Seek practitioners who are open to integrative medicine approaches. These professionals recognize the value of complementary therapies and are willing to discuss how they can fit into your treatment plan. Establishing mutual respect and understanding is vital. It fosters a partnership where you feel comfortable discussing your preferences and concerns, encouraging a more personalized and effective healthcare experience.

Understanding the role of each practitioner in your holistic health journey is essential. Your primary care physician acts as the cornerstone of your health management, monitoring overall well-being and coordinating care among specialists. They provide a broad perspective, ensuring all aspects of your health are considered. Specialists, on the other hand, offer expertise in specific areas, addressing particular health issues with focused attention. Their insights can be invaluable, especially when dealing with complex conditions. Holistic practitioners, such as acupuncturists or nutritionists, complement this team by providing therapies that support traditional treatments. Together, these professionals form a network of care that addresses the diverse needs of your body, mind, and spirit.

Navigating the healthcare system to ensure comprehensive care can be daunting, but with the right tools, it becomes manageable. Patient portals are invaluable resources, offering a centralized platform for communication with your healthcare team. They allow you to access medical records, schedule appointments, and message your providers, streamlining the management of your health information. Understanding your insurance coverage for integrative therapies is also crucial. Some policies cover complementary treatments like acupuncture or chiropractic care, while others may not. Reviewing your plan can help you make informed choices about your care options. Coordinating care among multiple providers requires clear communication. Ensure that each member of your healthcare team is aware of your entire treatment plan, fostering a unified approach to your health.

Reflective Exercise

Consider creating a health journal to record your experiences with integrative medicine. Document your holistic practices, medical treatments, and any changes in symptoms or well-being. This journal can serve as a valuable tool during medical appointments, helping you track progress and communicate effectively with your healthcare providers. Reflect on how different therapies impact your health, and note any questions or concerns that arise. By maintaining this record, you empower yourself to actively participate in your healthcare journey, fostering a deeper connection with your body and enhancing collaboration with your medical team.

The integration of conventional and complementary therapies offers a path to comprehensive care, one that honors the complexity of human health. By embracing this approach, you open yourself to a more holistic understanding of wellness, where every part of your being is nurtured and supported.

11.2 Complementary Therapies for Chronic Conditions

Living with a chronic condition often feels like navigating a complex maze, where every turn seems to present a new challenge. Conventional treatments provide relief, yet there remains a yearning for something more, a way to engage with the body and mind in a manner that feels holistic and nurturing. This is where complementary therapies come into play, offering additional paths to explore. Acupuncture, for instance, has gained recognition for its ability to alleviate pain and reduce inflammation. By gently inserting fine needles at specific points on the body, acupuncture aims to restore balance and promote the body's natural healing processes. Many patients report a decrease in pain and an increase in overall well-being following regular sessions. Chiropractic care, another valuable therapy, focuses on musculoskeletal issues. By adjusting the spine and other parts of the body, chiropractors aim to improve mobility and relieve pain. These adjustments can be particularly beneficial for individuals suffering from back pain, headaches, or joint discomfort. Meanwhile, massage therapy provides a sanctuary of relaxation, helping to reduce stress and tension. The therapeutic touch of massage can ease muscle tightness and promote circulation, fostering a sense of deep relaxation and rejuvenation.

Evaluating the effectiveness of these therapies is crucial to ensure they meet your personal health goals. Keeping a detailed symptom journal can be an invaluable tool in this process. By recording your symptoms before and after each session, you can track changes over time and identify patterns. This practice not only helps you assess the immediate impact of a therapy but also provides insights into longer-term benefits. Regular consultations with healthcare providers offer another layer of evaluation. Discuss your experiences with your doctor, sharing your symptom journal and any observations you have made. This collaboration allows for a comprehensive understanding of how the therapies are affecting you and helps in making informed decisions about continuing or adjusting treatments.

Tailoring complementary therapies to your individual needs involves a thoughtful approach. Each person is unique, and therapies that work for one individual may not work for another. Personalizing herbal therapy, for example, requires consideration of specific ailments and how different herbs might address them. A trained herbalist can help you select the right combinations, taking into account your health history and current condition. Similarly, adjusting the frequency of therapy sessions based on your response is essential. Some people may benefit from weekly sessions, while others might find that a less frequent schedule suits them better. Monitoring your progress and making adjustments as needed ensures that the therapies remain effective and supportive of your health goals.

Safety and precautions are paramount when engaging in complementary therapies. Ensuring that treatments are administered by certified practitioners is a fundamental step in safeguarding your health. Certified professionals have undergone rigorous training and adhere to standards that prioritize safety and efficacy. Being aware of potential side effects and interactions with medications is equally important. For instance, certain herbal supplements may interact with prescribed medications, altering their effectiveness or causing adverse reactions. Consult your healthcare provider before beginning any new therapy to discuss these potential interactions. This dialogue ensures that your healthcare team is fully aware of all treatments you are receiving and can provide guidance on how to integrate them safely into your overall care plan.

Understanding the landscape of complementary therapies can empower you to take an active role in managing chronic conditions. These therapies offer a chance to explore additional avenues of healing, complementing conventional treatments with practices that resonate with the body's natural rhythms. They invite you to engage with your health in a holistic manner, considering the physical, mental, and emotional aspects of well-being. The journey through this realm is not about replacing traditional medicine but enhancing it, creating a tapestry of care that is rich, diverse, and tailored to your unique needs. In the next chapter, we will explore the importance of self-care, delving into daily routines that nurture the body and mind, setting the stage for a life of balance and fulfillment.

Chapter 12
The Importance of Self-Care

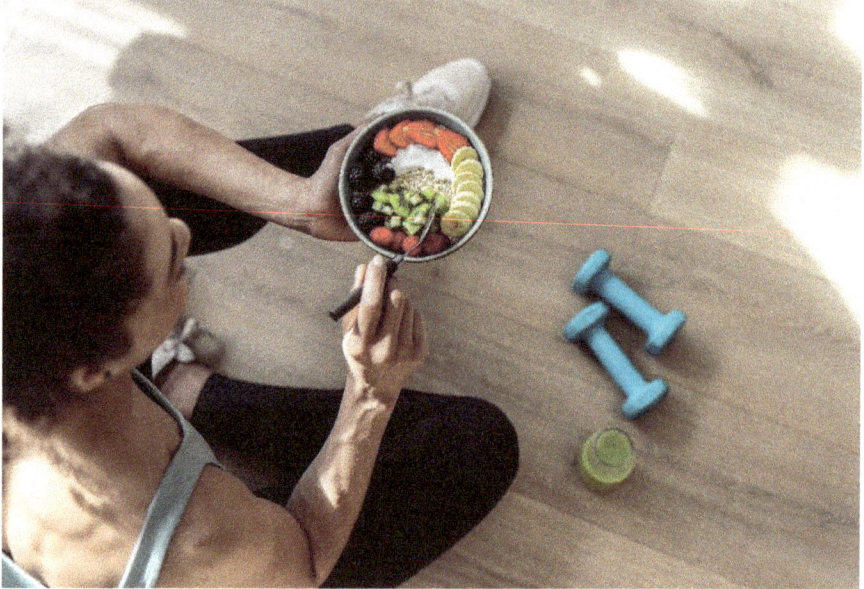

In the heart of a bustling city, amid the cacophony of honking horns and hurried footsteps, I found myself at a quaint coffee shop. It was one of those rare moments where time seemed to slow, and I could simply breathe. As I sipped my coffee, I realized how often I neglected these small moments of reprieve. This revelation, though simple, was profound. Self-care is not an indulgence; it's a necessity, much like that vital first breath of air each morning. This chapter explores the essence of self-care, demystifying its role in nurturing our mental, emotional, and physical health.

Self-care is often misinterpreted as a luxury, something to be indulged in only when time and resources allow. However, this couldn't be further from the truth. Self-care is about recognizing and tending to your needs, ensuring that you are well-equipped to face the demands of daily life. It's the foundation upon which mental clarity, emotional stability, and physical health are built. Differentiating self-care from self-indulgence is crucial. While self-care is intentional and restorative, self-indulgence often provides temporary relief without addressing underlying needs. Think of self-care as the maintenance required to keep a car running smoothly, rather than a fleeting joyride.

A robust self-care routine consists of key elements that harmonize with the rhythm of your day. Morning rituals set the tone, offering a positive start through activities like gentle stretching, a quiet moment of gratitude, or a nutritious breakfast. These practices awaken the senses, grounding you in the present and preparing you for the day ahead. As the sun sets, evening practices help you wind down, shedding the day's stress. This might involve reading, journaling, or a warm bath to soothe the soul. Throughout the day, moments of mindfulness act as anchors, allowing you to pause, breathe, and reconnect with yourself. These elements create a tapestry of care that supports you holistically.

Personalizing your self-care routine ensures that it resonates with your unique needs and preferences. It's about selecting activities that bring joy and fulfillment, whether that's painting, gardening, or practicing yoga. The beauty of self-care lies in its adaptability. Adjust your routines to accommodate your daily schedule, allowing space for spontaneity and flexibility. If mornings are hectic, perhaps a short evening meditation suits you better. The key is to listen to your body and mind, honoring what feels right in the moment.

Consistency in self-care is supported by various tools and resources. Planners or apps can track your self-care activities, providing structure and accountability. Apps like Aloe Bud offer gentle reminders to engage in daily self-care practices, while journaling apps encourage reflection and mindfulness. Setting reminders for scheduled self-care time ensures that these moments are prioritized amidst life's demands. Creating a dedicated self-care space at home, whether a cozy reading nook or a serene corner for meditation, reinforces the importance of these practices. This space serves as a refuge, a reminder that self-care is an integral part of your routine.

Self-Care Reflection Exercise

Consider taking a few minutes each week to reflect on your self-care practices. What activities have you enjoyed? Which ones felt most restorative? Use this reflection to adjust and refine your routine, ensuring it remains aligned with your needs. This exercise not only enhances self-awareness but also fosters a deeper connection with yourself, reminding you that self-care is a journey, not a destination.

12.1 The Role of Rest and Recovery

In the hustle and bustle of our daily lives, rest often takes a backseat. Yet, it's a cornerstone of self-care, vital for replenishing our energy reserves. Without adequate rest, our bodies struggle to repair and regenerate, leaving us vulnerable to fatigue and burnout. Rest is more than just sleep; it's a holistic approach to rejuvenation, crucial for maintaining both physical vitality and mental clarity. When we allow ourselves to pause, we give our bodies the chance to recover from the stresses of the day, and our minds the opportunity to reset. This replenishment is not a luxury but a necessity, akin to refueling a car that has traveled far and wide. Without it, we risk running on empty, which can lead to exhaustion and diminished well-being.

Understanding the different types of rest and recovery can transform how we recharge. Active rest, for instance, involves engaging in gentle activities that relax the body without exerting it. A leisurely walk in the park or a session of yoga can invigorate the senses while promoting relaxation. It's about finding activities that soothe rather than strain. Mental rest is equally important. In our digital age, our minds are constantly bombarded with information. Taking a break from screens through digital detoxes or meditation can quiet the mental noise. Meditation, in particular, provides a sanctuary for the mind, a space to breathe and be present. These restful practices allow us to step away from the chaos, giving our minds a much-needed respite. By embracing various forms of rest, we create a balanced approach to recovery that nurtures every aspect of our being.

Creating environments that promote rest is pivotal to enhancing our relaxation. A sleep-friendly bedroom is the foundation of restorative rest. Consider calming colors like soft blues or gentle greens that soothe the senses. Declutter the space to create a sense of tranquility; a cluttered room can lead to a cluttered mind. Introducing calming scents, such as lavender or chamomile, can further enhance relaxation. These scents have been shown to reduce anxiety and improve sleep quality. Simple additions like an essential oil diffuser or a lavender-scented pillow spray can transform your bedroom into a restful haven. These environmental adjustments act as subtle cues, signaling to your mind and body that it's time to unwind. By thoughtfully designing our spaces, we lay the groundwork for restful and rejuvenating experiences.

Incorporating recovery practices into daily life is essential for sustained well-being. One effective strategy is scheduling regular breaks throughout the workday. These breaks don't have to be long; even a few minutes to stretch or step outside can refresh the mind and body. Restorative yoga, practiced before bedtime, can also aid in winding down. This practice involves gentle poses that relax the body and prepare it for sleep. By stretching and breathing deeply, you release tension and promote a calm state of mind. Setting boundaries around personal time is another crucial aspect. In our hyper-connected world, it's easy to blur the lines between work and rest. Establish clear boundaries to protect your downtime, ensuring that you have uninterrupted periods for relaxation. This might involve turning off work notifications after hours or dedicating time each evening to unwind without distractions. These practices reinforce the importance of rest, integrating it into the fabric of daily life.

12.2 Setting Healthy Boundaries

Healthy boundaries are like invisible lines that define where your space begins and ends, allowing you to protect your well-being while engaging with the world. They're not barriers to keep others out but rather a form of self-respect and self-protection, ensuring that your needs and limits are acknowledged and respected. Think of boundaries as the framework of a house; they provide structure and security, allowing you to invite others in without losing your sense of self. Differentiating between rigid, porous, and healthy boundaries is crucial. Rigid boundaries act like walls, isolating you from meaningful connections, while porous boundaries are too permeable, leading to overcommitment and emotional exhaustion. Healthy boundaries, however, strike a balance, providing flexibility and strength, much like the gentle sway of a tree in the wind.

Identifying areas in your life where boundaries are needed is a reflective process that requires honest self-assessment. In the workplace, setting boundaries can prevent overcommitment and burnout. Perhaps you find yourself taking on extra tasks that stretch you thin, affecting your performance and well-being. Establishing clear limits on your workload and learning to say no when necessary can protect your professional integrity and mental health. Similarly, personal relationships demand boundaries to safeguard your emotional well-being. Consider the dynamics of your friendships and familial ties. Are there interactions that leave you feeling drained or unappreciated? Recognizing these patterns allows you to set boundaries that foster healthier and more fulfilling connections. By examining these areas, you gain clarity on where boundaries are needed, empowering you to create a life that honors your needs.

Establishing boundaries is a skill that involves clear communication and self-awareness. Practicing assertive communication techniques is a vital step in expressing your needs and limits. This doesn't mean being aggressive or confrontational; rather, it's about being clear and firm, respecting both yourself and others. Using "I" statements can effectively communicate your feelings and boundaries without placing blame. For example, saying, "I need some time to recharge after work, so I'll be unavailable for calls in the evening," clearly sets a limit while maintaining respect. These statements focus on your needs and experiences, allowing for open and honest dialogue. By articulating your boundaries assertively, you create an environment where they are more likely to be respected and understood.

Maintaining boundaries over time requires consistent effort and reflection. It's essential to regularly review and adjust your boundaries as your circumstances and needs evolve. Life is dynamic, and what worked in the past may no longer serve you. By revisiting your boundaries periodically, you ensure they remain relevant and effective. Challenges will inevitably arise, whether from external pressures or internal doubts. In such moments, seeking support from friends, counselors, or mentors can provide valuable perspective and encouragement. Their insights can help reinforce your commitment to your boundaries and offer strategies for overcoming obstacles. Consistency in actions and decisions is also key. By consistently upholding your boundaries, you reinforce their importance, making it easier for others to understand and respect them. This consistency fosters a sense of stability and confidence, allowing you to navigate life's complexities with greater ease and assurance.

As we conclude this chapter, remember that setting healthy boundaries is a continuous process that evolves with you. By understanding their importance and implementing them thoughtfully, you create a foundation for self-care and meaningful connections. Boundaries are not just about saying no; they are about saying yes to a life that reflects your values and needs. As we move forward, consider how these principles can enhance your journey towards holistic health, allowing you to engage with the world from a place of strength and clarity. In the next chapter, we will explore how holistic health practices can be integrated into community settings, further enriching our lives and those around us.

Chapter 13
Holistic Health and Community

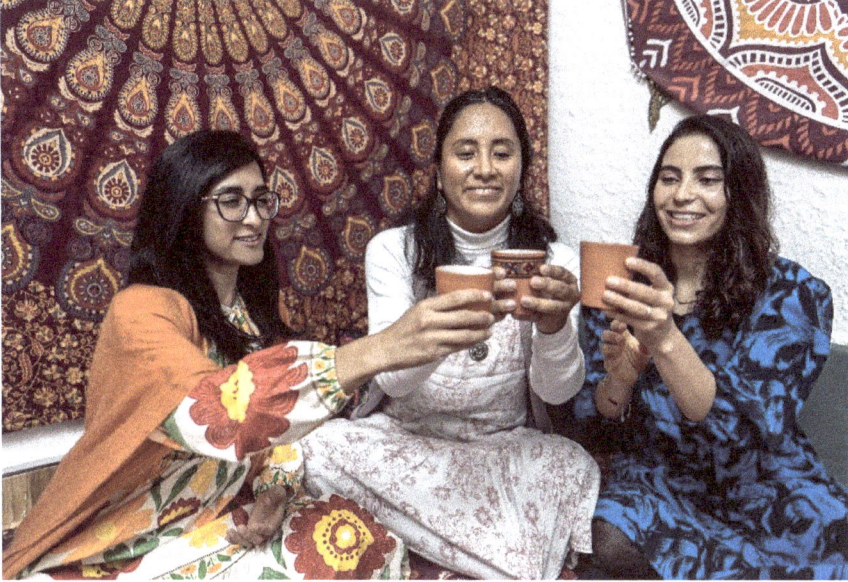

The world we navigate often feels vast and impersonal, yet within this expanse lies the potential for profound connection. Picture a quiet Saturday morning in a sunlit community hall. A group gathers, each individual bringing their own stories and hopes, united by a shared goal: embracing holistic health. There's an energy in the room, a palpable sense of purpose that transcends the ordinary. This scene encapsulates the essence of wellness communities, spaces where individuals come together, not just to improve their own health, but to uplift and support one another in a collective journey toward well-being.

13.1 Building Supportive Wellness Communities

A wellness community thrives on shared objectives and mutual support, creating an atmosphere where holistic health can flourish. At its core, a wellness community is a group of individuals committed to health and well-being, bound by common goals and a desire to foster a supportive environment. These communities emphasize the power of mutual support and accountability, recognizing that the journey to holistic health is more manageable when shared. Members encourage one another, celebrating successes and offering solace in times of struggle. This shared commitment cultivates a sense of belonging and camaraderie, transforming the pursuit of health from a solitary endeavor into a collective movement.

Being part of a wellness community offers numerous benefits, both tangible and intangible. Firstly, the sense of accountability inherent in these groups can significantly boost motivation, helping individuals adhere to health practices more consistently. When surrounded by others who share similar goals, the commitment to personal wellness becomes stronger. Additionally, wellness communities provide access to a diverse range of perspectives and experiences. Members bring their unique backgrounds and insights, enriching the collective knowledge of the group. This diversity fosters learning and growth, offering new strategies and ideas that may not have been considered individually. Moreover, the social connections forged within these communities can alleviate feelings of isolation, promoting emotional well-being and resilience.

Creating and sustaining a wellness community requires thoughtful planning and ongoing effort. Organizing regular community events is crucial for maintaining engagement and fostering a sense of unity. These events can take various forms, from yoga classes and meditation sessions to health workshops and discussion groups. They provide opportunities for members to connect, share experiences, and learn from one another. Utilizing social media platforms can also enhance community engagement, allowing members to stay connected and informed even when apart. Online wellness groups provide a space for discussion, resource sharing, and encouragement, bridging the gap between in-person meetings. Encouraging collaborative projects and initiatives further strengthens the community, promoting a sense of ownership and investment among members.

Despite the many advantages, building a wellness community presents challenges that must be navigated with care. Differing opinions and conflicts may arise, as members bring diverse perspectives and backgrounds. It's essential to foster an environment of respect and open communication, where differences can be discussed constructively. Establishing clear guidelines and facilitating discussions with empathy and understanding can help manage these challenges. Sustaining engagement over time requires creativity and adaptability. Regularly evaluating and refreshing community activities can keep members engaged and motivated. Encouraging member feedback and involvement in decision-making processes ensures that the community remains dynamic and responsive to its members' needs.

Reflection Exercise: Building Your Wellness Community

Take a moment to envision the wellness community you aspire to create or join. Consider the goals, activities, and values that resonate with you. Reflect on the steps needed to bring this vision to life. What skills or resources can you contribute? How can you engage and inspire others to join this collective pursuit of holistic health? Write down your thoughts and ideas, creating a blueprint for your wellness community. This exercise can guide your efforts, providing clarity and motivation as you embark on building a supportive network dedicated to holistic well-being.

In embracing the concept of wellness communities, you tap into a powerful resource for personal and collective growth. These communities offer more than just support; they provide a platform for transformation, where individuals can explore holistic health in a nurturing and collaborative environment. As you engage with others in this shared journey, you not only enhance your own well-being but contribute to a larger movement toward balanced living and inner peace.

13.2 Family Involvement in Holistic Practices

Family dynamics play a crucial role in shaping our health practices and outcomes. They provide a backdrop of support and influence that can either propel us toward wellness or hinder our progress. Picture a family dinner table where discussions flow as freely as the food, where encouragement and understanding form the basis of every meal. In such settings, emotional support from family members becomes a cornerstone of holistic health. When family members cheer each other on, they create an environment of safety and encouragement. This emotional foundation makes it easier to adopt new health habits, knowing that every step is met with understanding and support. Moreover, family habits and routines exert a profound impact on personal health choices. The daily rituals we share with our loved ones, whether it's a morning walk, a shared meal, or an evening meditation, can significantly shape our approach to health. These routines offer a framework upon which individual practices are built, demonstrating the powerful role family plays in holistic health.

Integrating holistic practices into family life enhances not only individual well-being but also the collective health of the family unit. Start with family meal planning, emphasizing whole foods and balanced nutrition. Inviting everyone to participate in planning and preparing meals fosters a sense of ownership and responsibility. Choose vibrant vegetables, lean proteins, and whole grains as the staples of your meals. Consider setting a family goal to try a new healthy recipe each week. This not only diversifies your diet but also provides a fun and engaging activity for the whole family. Beyond the kitchen, incorporating group mindfulness activities can bring family members closer while promoting mental well-being. Regular meditation sessions or nature walks offer moments of shared tranquility, allowing everyone to unwind and connect. These activities can be simple yet impactful, providing a space for reflection and bonding. By weaving these practices into your daily routine, you create a holistic environment that nurtures both body and spirit.

Engaging family members of all ages in holistic practices fosters a sense of unity and inclusivity. Tailor activities to suit varying ages and abilities, ensuring that everyone can participate and benefit. For younger children, interactive activities like gardening or yoga can be both educational and enjoyable. Teenagers might appreciate more challenging pursuits like hiking or team sports, which encourage physical activity and social interaction. For older family members, gentle exercises like tai chi or chair yoga can promote flexibility and balance. Consider creating intergenerational wellness challenges or goals that encourage collaboration and teamwork. Whether it's a monthly step count challenge or a commitment to practicing gratitude daily, these goals can motivate family members to support one another in their pursuits. These shared experiences not only promote physical health but also strengthen family bonds, creating lasting memories and traditions.

Addressing resistance and building consensus within the family is essential for fostering a supportive environment. Open communication about the benefits of holistic practices is key to overcoming skepticism or reluctance. Share personal experiences or stories that highlight the positive impact of holistic health, emphasizing how these practices can enhance everyone's quality of life. Involve family members in decision-making and goal-setting, ensuring that their voices and preferences are heard. This collaborative approach fosters a sense of autonomy and respect, making it easier to reach a consensus. Celebrate small achievements and progress together, acknowledging the effort and dedication of each family member. Whether it's a healthier meal choice, a successful meditation session, or a completed fitness milestone, celebrating these moments reinforces the value of holistic practices and encourages continued participation.

In embracing holistic practices as a family, you create a nurturing environment that supports collective well-being. The family becomes a source of strength and inspiration, where shared goals and experiences enrich each member's journey toward health. As you navigate this path together, you build a foundation of wellness that extends beyond the individual, fostering a sense of harmony and connection within the family unit.

As we continue this exploration of holistic health, the next chapter will delve into affordable holistic practices, offering practical tips and strategies for integrating wellness into everyday life.

Chapter 14
Affordable Holistic Practices

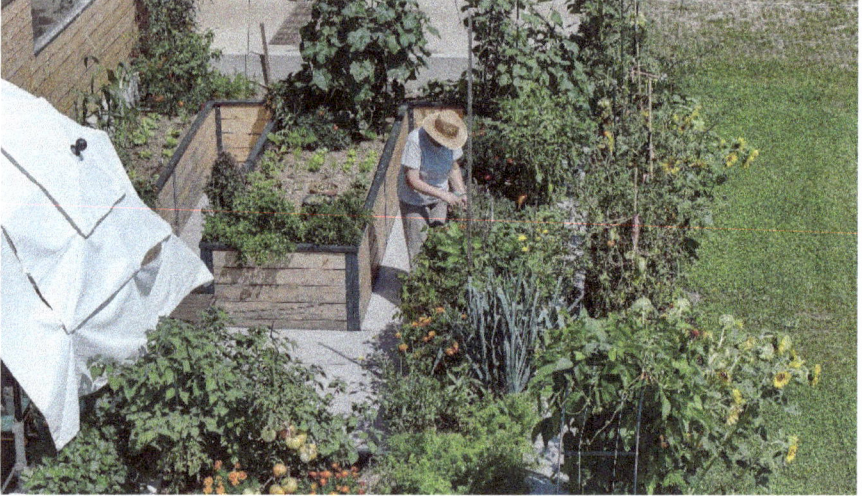

In the heart of a bustling city, I once found myself captivated by a small herbal shop tucked between towering buildings. The shop owner, an elderly woman with a wealth of knowledge, shared with me age-old remedies crafted from common household ingredients. Her stories of healing inspired me to explore the world of do-it-yourself (DIY) remedies, which offer an accessible and personalized approach to health. In today's fast-paced world, where convenience often trumps tradition, these natural solutions provide a refreshing alternative. They empower you to take control of your health using ingredients already in your pantry, offering not just remedies but a deeper connection to the natural world.

14.1 DIY Remedies for Common Ailments

Creating DIY remedies at home is a simple yet powerful practice that transforms everyday ingredients into potent allies for health. The beauty of these remedies lies in their accessibility and personalization. You save money by using items you already have, avoiding the expense of over-the-counter medications. Moreover, you can tailor these remedies to suit your personal preferences and sensitivities, ensuring they align with your unique needs. This approach allows for creativity and experimentation, enabling you to discover what works best for you. By crafting your own remedies, you engage in a form of self-care that fosters a sense of empowerment and autonomy over your health.

One of the most cherished DIY remedies for soothing a sore throat is a honey and lemon syrup. Honey, with its natural antibacterial properties, coats and soothes the throat, while lemon provides a burst of vitamin C, supporting the immune system. To prepare, simply mix a tablespoon of honey with the juice of half a lemon in a cup of warm water. Sip slowly, allowing the syrup to coat your throat, providing relief and comfort. Another reliable remedy is ginger tea, renowned for its ability to ease nausea and support digestion. Ginger's anti-inflammatory properties make it a powerful ingredient for calming an upset stomach. To make ginger tea, peel and slice a small piece of fresh ginger, add it to a pot of boiling water, and let it simmer for about 10 minutes. Strain the tea into a cup, and add honey or lemon for extra flavor and benefits. These simple remedies harness nature's power to promote healing and well-being.

Crafting your own remedies at home is a rewarding process, but it's essential to follow safe practices to ensure effectiveness and safety. Take, for instance, the soothing oatmeal bath for irritated skin. Begin by blending a cup of plain oatmeal into a fine powder and adding it to a warm bath. The oatmeal's natural properties will soothe and moisturize the skin, providing relief from irritation. For a homemade vapor rub, combine a carrier oil like coconut oil with a few drops of eucalyptus and peppermint essential oils. These oils, known for their decongestant properties, can relieve congestion when applied to the chest. Mix well and store in a small jar, and remember to apply sparingly, as a little goes a long way.

Safety is paramount when using DIY remedies, and there are several precautions to keep in mind. Always conduct a patch test before using a new remedy, especially those involving essential oils, to ensure you do not have any allergic reactions. Apply a small amount of the mixture to your skin and wait 24 hours to check for any irritation. Proper storage is also crucial to maintain the potency and shelf life of your homemade concoctions. Store them in airtight containers, away from direct sunlight and extreme temperatures. This protects the ingredients and ensures they remain safe and effective for use. By following these guidelines, you can enjoy the benefits of DIY remedies with confidence and peace of mind.

DIY Remedy Checklist

- Identify the ailment you wish to address.
- Select the appropriate ingredients, ensuring they are fresh and high-quality.
- Follow step-by-step instructions to prepare the remedy safely.
- Conduct a patch test for new ingredients.
- Store the remedy in a suitable container, labeled with the preparation date.

DIY remedies offer a holistic approach to health, blending tradition with practicality. They invite you to explore the healing potential of nature, crafting solutions that are both effective and tailored to your needs.

14.2 Free Online Resources for Wellness

In today's digital age, the internet is a goldmine of resources for those seeking to enhance their holistic health practices without spending a dime. One of the most accessible platforms is YouTube, where you can find a plethora of guided yoga and meditation sessions tailored to all levels of experience. Whether you're a beginner looking to learn the basics or someone seeking advanced techniques, YouTube has something for you. Many instructors offer free classes that you can follow at your own pace, allowing you to practice in the comfort of your home. The convenience of pausing, rewinding, or replaying sessions as needed makes it an ideal tool for fitting wellness activities into your schedule. Additionally, you can explore wellness forums, which provide a community of like-minded individuals ready to offer support and share advice. These forums are invaluable for those who seek human connection and encouragement on their path to better health. You can exchange ideas, ask questions, and learn from the experiences of others, building a network of support that enriches your wellness journey.

Educational content is another treasure trove available online, supporting your learning and practice in holistic health. Health podcasts are a fantastic way to gain expert insights while on the go. You can listen during your commute, workout, or even while cooking, turning everyday activities into opportunities for growth. These podcasts often feature interviews with health professionals, offering diverse perspectives on wellness topics. Additionally, reputable wellness websites offer a wealth of e-books and articles, presenting in-depth information on various aspects of holistic health. These resources are often crafted by experts in the field, ensuring you receive quality information to guide your practice. Reading these materials helps you stay informed about the latest health trends and research, empowering you to make educated decisions about your wellness practices.

Wellness apps have revolutionized how we manage and track our health practices, providing tools that fit right into our pockets. Meditation apps like Insight Timer offer free guided sessions, catering to different meditation styles and durations. They often include features like progress tracking and reminders, helping you cultivate a consistent practice. The ability to choose sessions based on mood or goal allows for a personalized experience, making meditation more accessible and enjoyable. Nutrition trackers are equally beneficial, providing a simple way to monitor dietary habits and ensure balanced nutrition. These apps can help you set goals, track caloric intake, and even suggest healthier food alternatives, supporting your efforts to maintain a nutritious diet. By leveraging these apps, you can streamline your wellness routine, making it easier to incorporate healthy habits into your daily life.

Finally, building online wellness networks can significantly enhance your holistic health journey. Social media groups centered around wellness topics offer platforms for sharing experiences, challenges, and triumphs. Engaging with these communities provides a sense of belonging and accountability, vital for sustaining motivation. Whether participating in discussions or simply observing, these interactions can inspire and inform your practices. Virtual wellness challenges and activities are another exciting way to stay engaged. These challenges often involve group goals, such as a month-long meditation streak or a healthy eating challenge, fostering a spirit of camaraderie and support. By joining these networks, you tap into a collective energy that propels you toward your wellness goals, enriching your holistic health experience in ways that are both meaningful and accessible.

14.3 Budget-Friendly Nutrition Hacks

Navigating the aisles of a grocery store with a mindful eye can transform the way you shop. Buying in bulk is a strategy that can significantly cut costs on staple foods like grains and beans. These items are not only versatile but also have a long shelf life, making them ideal for bulk purchases. Imagine the possibilities with a large bag of rice or a sack of dried beans; they can be the foundation for countless hearty meals. Similarly, choosing seasonal produce is another savvy way to save money while enjoying peak freshness and flavor. Seasonal fruits and vegetables are often less expensive because they are abundant, and their quality is unmatched by off-season imports. Walking through a farmers' market, you'll find the vibrancy of local, in-season produce not just appealing to the eye but also to the wallet.

Effective meal planning is another key to stretching your budget while reducing food waste. By creating weekly meal plans based on available deals and discounts, you can ensure that you're getting the most value for your money. This approach allows you to plan your meals around what's on sale, rather than impulse buying. Consider setting aside time each week to scan grocery store flyers or use apps that highlight weekly specials. Moreover, utilizing leftovers creatively can minimize waste and save you from unnecessary spending. For instance, roasted vegetables from dinner can become the star of a lunchtime salad the next day. Leftover chicken can be transformed into a flavorful soup or stir-fry, making meal planning both economical and exciting.

Incorporating superfoods into your diet doesn't have to strain your budget. Lentils, for example, are an affordable and protein-rich option that can be used in a variety of dishes. From hearty stews to refreshing salads, lentils provide essential nutrients while being gentle on the wallet. Cabbage and kale are also cost-effective superfoods, packed with vitamins and minerals. These nutrient-dense vegetables are incredibly versatile, suitable for salads, soups, or stir-fries. Their robust flavors and textures can elevate any dish, making them a staple in budget-conscious kitchens. By focusing on these affordable superfoods, you're investing in both your health and your financial well-being.

Cooking economically doesn't mean sacrificing flavor or nutrition. One-pot meals are a fantastic way to minimize ingredients while maximizing flavor. These dishes often involve combining grains, proteins, and vegetables in a single pot, allowing flavors to meld beautifully. Imagine a fragrant curry simmering on the stove, its rich aroma filling your kitchen, or a comforting stew that warms you from the inside out. Slow-cooker recipes are equally beneficial, offering hearty and budget-friendly dinners with minimal effort. Simply add your ingredients in the morning, and by evening, you'll have a delicious meal ready to enjoy. These cooking methods not only save money but also time, making them perfect for busy individuals who still want to eat well.

DIY nutrition enhancers are another way to boost your meals without breaking the bank. Making homemade nut butters and spreads is a simple project that can add both flavor and nutrition to your diet. By blending nuts with a touch of salt or honey, you create a delicious spread that rivals store-bought versions in taste and quality. Growing herbs on windowsills provides fresh seasoning at your fingertips, elevating your dishes with vibrant flavors. Basil, rosemary, and mint are just a few examples of herbs that thrive indoors, offering a touch of green to your home and a burst of freshness to your meals. These DIY projects not only enhance your nutrition but also add a personal touch to your culinary creations.

Chapter 15
Cultural Inclusivity in Holistic Practices

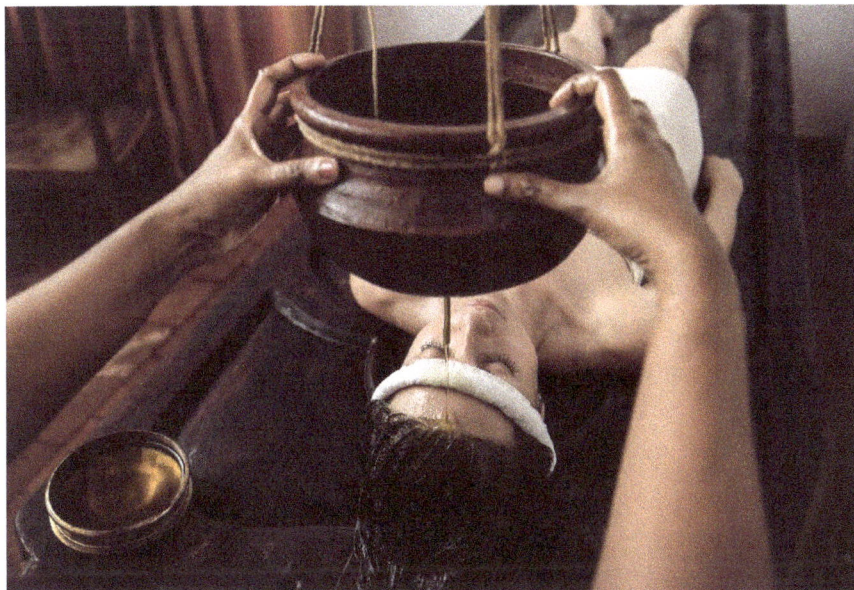

Imagine a world where ancient wisdom meets modern understanding, where practices honed over centuries come alive in the bustling kitchens and tranquil living rooms of our contemporary lives. Such is the world of Ayurveda, an ancient Indian system of medicine that continues to offer profound insights into health and well-being. My first encounter with Ayurveda came during a visit to Kerala, India, a region renowned for its traditional healing techniques. There, amidst the lush greenery and gentle rhythms of daily life, I witnessed the harmony of Ayurveda in action. Local practitioners used time-honored methods to treat ailments, emphasizing balance and personal constitution. This experience opened my eyes to the power of Ayurveda and its potential to enrich our modern lives.

Ayurveda, often translated as "the science of life," is one of the world's oldest holistic healing systems, with roots stretching back over 3,000 years. It is based on the belief that health and wellness depend on a delicate balance between the mind, body, and spirit. According to

Ayurveda, every individual is unique, and understanding one's constitution, or Prakriti, is key to maintaining health. Prakriti is determined by the balance of three fundamental energies known as doshas: Vata, Pitta, and Kapha. Vata governs movement and is associated with qualities like lightness and flexibility. Pitta controls transformation, linked to heat and intensity. Kapha manages structure and stability, characterized by heaviness and endurance. Each person has a distinct combination of these doshas, which influences their physical characteristics, mental traits, and tendencies toward certain health conditions. Discovering your dosha can provide valuable insights into your health, guiding you toward personalized wellness.

Incorporating Ayurvedic practices into daily life can promote balance and enhance well-being. One foundational practice is Dinacharya, a set of daily routines designed to align with natural rhythms and support dosha balance. These routines might include waking up early, practicing meditation, and eating meals at consistent times. Dinacharya fosters harmony in the body and mind, creating a sense of stability. Abhyanga, or self-massage with warm oil, is another cherished Ayurvedic practice. The oils used in Abhyanga are selected based on one's dosha and are believed to detoxify the body, improve circulation, and calm the nervous system. This soothing ritual can be a nurturing addition to your morning or evening routine. Nasya, a nasal cleansing technique, involves the application of herbal oils or ghee into the nostrils. It is said to enhance respiratory health, clear sinuses, and sharpen the senses. These practices, when tailored to your individual needs, can bring balance and vitality to your life.

Ayurvedic dietary principles emphasize the importance of eating according to your dosha type and the changing seasons. This approach acknowledges that our bodies have different needs throughout the year and that aligning our diet with these cycles can support health. For example, someone with a Vata constitution might benefit from warm, grounding foods like soups and stews during the cold months, while a Pitta individual might thrive on cooling foods like fresh vegetables and fruits in the summer. Central to Ayurvedic nutrition is the concept of Agni, or digestive fire, which is considered the root of all health. A strong Agni ensures efficient digestion, absorption, and assimilation of nutrients, while a weak Agni can lead to imbalances and disease. Ayurvedic guidelines suggest eating mindfully, favoring freshly prepared meals, and avoiding overeating to maintain a robust Agni. These principles encourage a balanced diet that nourishes both the body and the mind.

Ayurveda also offers a rich pharmacopeia of herbs and remedies, each with specific health benefits. Turmeric, a golden spice revered in Ayurvedic medicine, is celebrated for its potent anti-inflammatory properties. It has been used to support joint health, enhance digestion, and boost the immune system. Ashwagandha, an adaptogenic herb, is known for its ability to reduce stress and anxiety, promoting calmness and mental clarity. It is often recommended for those dealing with the pressures of modern life. Triphala, a traditional herbal blend, is valued for its detoxifying and digestive benefits. It consists of three fruits that work synergistically to cleanse the digestive tract, support regularity, and nourish the body. These herbs exemplify the holistic nature of Ayurveda, addressing health on multiple levels.

Reflection Section: Discovering Your Dosha

To begin your Ayurvedic journey, consider exploring your dosha type. Numerous online quizzes and resources can guide you in identifying your primary dosha. Reflect on your physical characteristics, mental traits, and health tendencies. Understanding your unique constitution can provide a roadmap for personalized wellness practices. Embrace this exploration as a step toward greater self-awareness and balance.

15.1 Traditional Chinese Medicine Approaches

Traditional Chinese Medicine (TCM) presents a fascinating perspective on health, emphasizing the vital force known as Qi, which flows through the body. This concept of Qi is central to TCM, seen as the life energy that fuels our physical and mental activities. When Qi flows freely, harmony prevails, and health is maintained. However, blockages or imbalances can lead to illness. In TCM, maintaining the balance of Yin and Yang, the complementary forces that represent opposite yet interconnected energies, is crucial. Yin embodies qualities like coolness, passivity, and darkness, while Yang represents warmth, activity, and light. Health depends on a dynamic equilibrium between these forces. The Five Elements, Wood, Fire, Earth, Metal, and Water, offer another layer to understanding the body's functions, each element correlating with specific organs and emotions. For instance, Wood is linked to the liver and anger, while Metal corresponds to the lungs and grief. These elements interact in complex ways, influencing health and well-being.

Acupuncture and acupressure are among the most recognized practices in TCM, celebrated for their ability to restore balance and promote healing. Acupuncture involves the insertion of thin needles into specific points on the body, aimed at unblocking Qi and restoring harmony. Common acupuncture points for stress relief and energy balance include those located on the ears, hands, and feet, areas rich in nerve endings and energy pathways. These points, when stimulated, can help alleviate tension, reduce stress, and enhance overall vitality. Acupressure, a related practice, applies pressure to these same points using fingers or special tools, offering a non-invasive alternative. It is particularly effective for treating headaches and tension, providing relief by encouraging the flow of Qi without needles. Many individuals find self-acupressure a useful tool for managing daily stress, as it can be performed anywhere and requires no special equipment.

Herbal medicine plays a significant role in TCM, using natural substances to support health and address specific ailments. Ginseng is one of the most well-known herbs, renowned for its ability to boost energy and bolster the immune system. It is often used to combat fatigue and enhance mental clarity. Ginger, another staple, is treasured for its digestive benefits, aiding in the relief of nausea and promoting healthy digestion. Its warming properties make it particularly beneficial for those with cold-related digestive issues. Goji berries, vibrant and nutrient-rich, are valued for their potential to support eye health and enhance vitality. They are often consumed as a snack or brewed into teas, providing a sweet, tangy boost to one's diet. These herbs, among others, form a cornerstone of TCM's holistic approach, offering natural solutions that align with the body's rhythms.

Movement practices like Qigong and Tai Chi are integral to TCM, focusing on cultivating and balancing Qi through physical exercise. Qigong, which translates to "skillful movement of life energy," involves gentle, flowing movements paired with mindful breathing. These exercises enhance the flow of Qi, promoting relaxation and vitality. Practitioners often report feeling more centered and energized after a session, as the movements encourage a meditative state. Tai Chi, often described as "meditation in motion," is characterized by its slow, deliberate movements that improve balance and coordination. This practice not only strengthens the body but also calms the mind, making it a valuable tool for stress reduction and overall well-being. Both Qigong and Tai Chi can be adapted to suit individual needs and fitness levels, offering accessible options for anyone interested in exploring TCM's movement practices.

Traditional Chinese Medicine's holistic approach to health emphasizes the interconnectedness of mind, body, and spirit. By maintaining the flow of Qi and balancing Yin and Yang, one can achieve harmony and well-being. Acupuncture, acupressure, herbal medicine, Qigong, and Tai Chi all contribute to TCM's comprehensive toolkit, offering diverse paths to health. These practices invite you to explore new avenues of self-care and healing, integrating ancient wisdom into modern life. As we move forward in this exploration of cultural inclusivity in holistic practices, consider how these principles might resonate with your personal health journey. The next chapter will delve into practical transformation stories, illustrating how holistic health can profoundly impact lives.

Chapter 16
Practical Transformation Stories

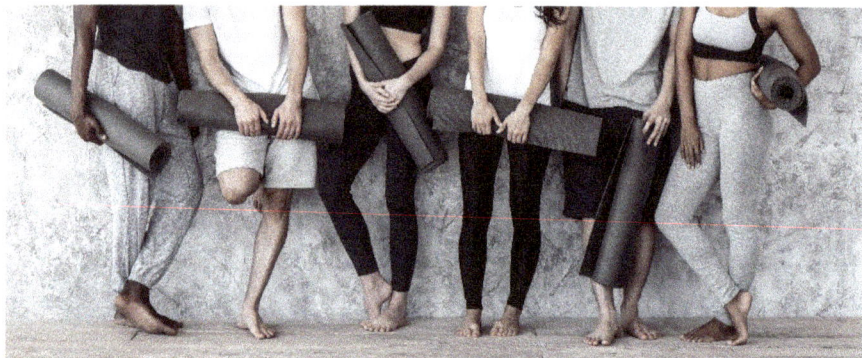

Imagine standing at the base of a steep hill, burdened by the weight of chronic pain that clings to you like a shadow. The road to relief seems distant, yet the promise of a pain-free life beckons from the summit. This is a journey that many embark upon, seeking solace in the embrace of holistic health. Let me share with you three inspiring stories of individuals who dared to traverse this path, overcoming their pain by embracing holistic practices that transformed their lives.

Sarah, a dedicated school teacher, found herself trapped in a cycle of chronic back pain that no amount of medication seemed to alleviate. Her days were punctuated by discomfort, and her nights were restless. Conventional pain management strategies offered little relief, often leaving her frustrated and disheartened. In her search for an alternative, she stumbled upon the practice of mindfulness meditation. Initially skeptical, she hesitated to embrace a method that seemed so intangible compared to the physicality of her pain. Yet, as she delved deeper into the practice, she discovered its profound impact. The body scan technique, where one focuses on each part of their body, became a cornerstone of her daily routine. This practice, outlined by Jon Kabat-Zinn and recommended by Harvard Health, taught her to observe her pain without judgment, reducing the stress it caused (SOURCE 1). With time, meditation became a powerful tool in her arsenal, allowing her to manage her pain more effectively.

Sarah's journey didn't stop at meditation. She began incorporating gentle yoga poses into her daily routine, focusing on those that promoted flexibility and strength without exacerbating her pain. Poses like the cat-cow and child's pose became her refuge, offering relief and comfort. The consistency of her practice, coupled with the support of a local yoga community, played a pivotal role in her recovery. Surrounded by individuals who understood her struggles and celebrated her progress, Sarah found the strength to persevere. Her journey is a testament to the power of the mind-body connection and the potential for transformation through holistic practices.

James, a software engineer, faced a different kind of battle. Chronic migraines had become an unwelcome part of his life, disrupting his work and personal life. Initially, he viewed acupuncture with skepticism, dismissing it as an unproven alternative to conventional treatments. However, the persistent nature of his migraines led him to reconsider. Encouraged by studies highlighting acupuncture's effectiveness in managing migraines (SOURCE 2), James decided to give it a chance. Under the guidance of a skilled practitioner, he embarked on a series of sessions that gradually reduced the frequency and intensity of his migraines. The needles, once feared, became symbols of hope and healing.

Alongside acupuncture, James made significant dietary changes, focusing on anti-inflammatory foods. He incorporated more fruits, vegetables, and omega-3-rich foods into his meals while reducing processed foods and sugars. These changes, though gradual, contributed to his overall well-being, complementing the effects of acupuncture. Over time, the combination of these practices not only alleviated his migraines but also enhanced his energy levels and mood. James's story underscores the importance of openness to new approaches and the transformative power of holistic nutrition.

Emma, a retired librarian, grappled with arthritis, a condition that left her joints swollen and painful. Traditional treatments offered limited relief, prompting her to explore herbal remedies. With the guidance of a knowledgeable herbalist, Emma began incorporating specific herbs into her routine. Turmeric, renowned for its anti-inflammatory properties, became a staple in her diet (SOURCE 3). She also embraced boswellia, a herbal supplement known for its ability to reduce inflammation and pain. These natural remedies, combined with gentle movement and stretching, started to make a noticeable difference.

Emma's daily routine evolved to include regular walks and gentle exercises designed to maintain joint mobility. She also embraced the practice of yoga, adapting poses to suit her comfort and capabilities. The support and advice from her herbalist were invaluable, providing tailored guidance that ensured her journey was both safe and effective. Emma's success story highlights the potential of herbal supplements and lifestyle modifications in managing arthritis pain. Her experience serves as a reminder of the importance of collaboration with healthcare professionals to achieve optimal results.

Reflection Section: Embracing Holistic Modalities

Think about your own health challenges and consider how holistic practices might fit into your life. Reflect on the stories of Sarah, James, and Emma, and identify elements that resonate with you. What steps can you take to explore the mind-body connection, nutrition, or herbal remedies? Write down your thoughts and create a plan to incorporate these practices into your routine. This reflection can serve as a guide to embarking on your own path to holistic health.

The stories of these chronic pain warriors reveal key lessons in the realm of holistic health. They demonstrate the value of exploring multiple modalities, acknowledging that healing is often a multifaceted process. Perseverance and patience emerge as vital components of their journeys, reminding us that transformation is rarely immediate but always possible. These narratives inspire us to seek personalized solutions, tailored to our unique needs and circumstances, and to embrace the holistic approach as a pathway to healing and well-being.

16.1 Transformative Weight Management Journeys

In the realm of weight management, Michael's story is one of resilience and transformation. For years, he found himself caught in the cycle of fad diets, each promising quick results but delivering only temporary changes. He would lose weight rapidly, only to gain it back just as quickly, leaving him frustrated and disheartened. These diets, often restrictive and unsustainable, took a toll on his physical and emotional well-being. It was during this time of disillusionment that Michael stumbled upon the concept of mindful eating. Instead of focusing on deprivation, he began to tune into his body's hunger and fullness cues. This shift marked a turning point in his approach to food and nutrition. Michael embraced whole foods, opting for meals rich in nutrients rather than empty calories. This mindful approach extended to portion control, allowing him to enjoy a variety of foods without the guilt associated with overeating.

In addition to changing his eating habits, Michael incorporated regular physical activity into his routine. He discovered the benefits of both aerobic exercises, like brisk walking and cycling, and strength training, which helped him build muscle and increase his metabolism. These activities not only contributed to his weight loss but also improved his overall fitness and energy levels. As he shed the pounds, Michael noticed a significant improvement in his mental and emotional health. The regular exercise released endorphins, elevating his mood and reducing stress. With each step forward, he felt a renewed sense of confidence and self-worth, proving that weight management is as much about mental resilience as it is about physical change.

Sophia's story highlights the power of community support in achieving weight management goals. She embarked on her journey with the help of a local wellness group, where she found camaraderie and encouragement. This group became a lifeline, providing a space where she could share her struggles and celebrate her successes. The shared experiences and mutual support kept her motivated, even when the path seemed challenging. In this supportive environment, Sophia learned the value of accountability. Her peers acted as both cheerleaders and mentors, offering advice and encouragement when needed. This sense of belonging instilled a sense of purpose and commitment in Sophia, driving her to stay consistent in her efforts.

Sophia also benefited from the personalized guidance of a holistic nutritionist. This professional helped her tailor a nutrition plan that suited her lifestyle and health goals. Together, they focused on balanced meals that included a variety of nutrients, ensuring that Sophia's body received the nourishment it needed. The nutritionist also introduced her to mindful eating practices, reinforcing the importance of listening to her body's signals. This personalized approach empowered Sophia to make informed choices, transforming her relationship with food into one of nourishment and enjoyment.

Lydia's journey offers a refreshing perspective on weight management, one that transcends the numbers on the scale. Her focus was not solely on losing weight but on enhancing her overall well-being. Lydia recognized the importance of mental health in her journey, committing to practices that supported her emotional resilience. She incorporated journaling into her daily routine, using it as a tool for self-reflection and emotional expression. This practice provided a safe space for Lydia to explore her thoughts and feelings, fostering a deeper understanding of her motivations and challenges. Meditation became another cornerstone of her routine, offering moments of peace and clarity amidst the hustle of daily life. These practices, though subtle, contributed significantly to Lydia's sense of balance and fulfillment.

Intuitive eating played a crucial role in Lydia's transformation, allowing her to foster a positive relationship with food. She embraced the principles of honoring her hunger, respecting her fullness, and savoring her meals without guilt. This approach liberated her from the constraints of dieting, encouraging her to trust her body's innate wisdom. Lydia's focus on well-being rather than weight alone resulted in a more sustainable and enjoyable lifestyle. As she tuned into her body's needs, she found that her energy levels improved, her mood stabilized, and her self-esteem soared.

The stories of Michael, Sophia, and Lydia reveal key insights into the holistic approach to weight management. They highlight the importance of considering mental and emotional health alongside physical changes. Michael's experience underscores the transformative power of mindful eating and consistent physical activity. Sophia's success demonstrates the impact of community support and personalized guidance. Lydia's journey emphasizes the value of nurturing a positive relationship with food and embracing practices that enhance overall well-being. Together, these narratives remind us that weight management is a multifaceted endeavor, one that requires a holistic mindset and a commitment to personal growth. As we continue to explore the path to holistic health, these stories serve as beacons of inspiration and hope.

Chapter 17
Measuring Holistic Health Success

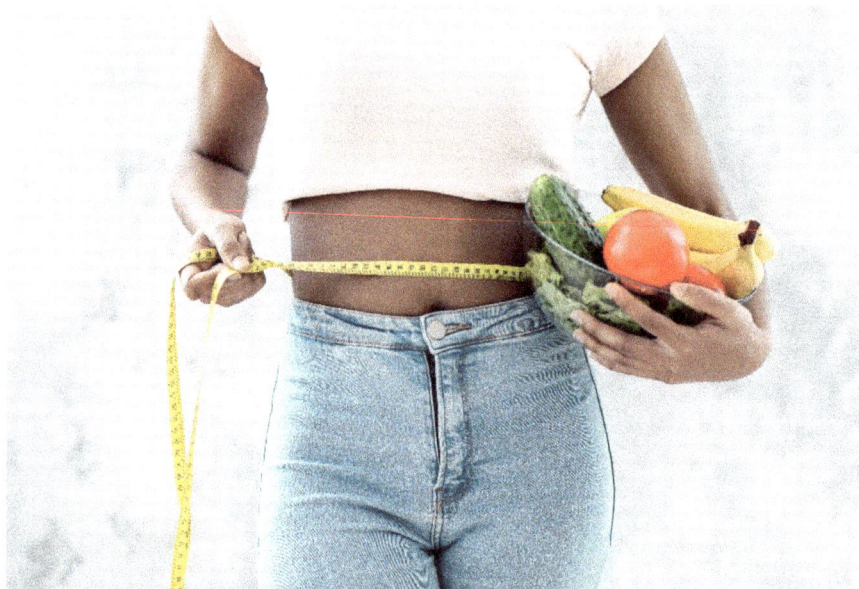

Imagine waking up one morning, deciding to embark on a journey toward better health, and finding yourself overwhelmed with where to begin. This is a common experience for many who set out to improve their physical well-being. I once met a patient who, despite being active, felt lost in the myriad of health advice and endless data. We worked together to identify clear, measurable physical health metrics that guided his progress. This chapter will illuminate the key indicators of physical health, empowering you to track and celebrate your achievements in a holistic journey.

17.1 Tracking Physical Health Improvements

When considering physical health, it's crucial to focus on metrics that truly reflect your well-being. Monitoring vital signs such as blood pressure and heart rate provides a window into cardiovascular health. These indicators can reveal stress levels and overall heart function, offering a baseline to build upon. Body composition, including muscle mass and fat percentage, further illustrates your fitness. Unlike weight alone, this metric highlights the balance between lean tissue and fat, offering a nuanced view of health. Flexibility and mobility, assessed through range-of-motion tests, indicate joint health and the ability to perform everyday tasks with ease. Endurance and cardiovascular fitness, evaluated through stamina tests, measure how well your body delivers oxygen during prolonged activity, reflecting heart and lung health.

In this digital age, technology plays a pivotal role in health tracking. Wearable fitness trackers have become ubiquitous, offering insights into steps taken, heart rate, and even sleep patterns. Devices like the Fitbit Charge 5 and Apple Watch Series 8 provide comprehensive data, enhancing motivation and accountability. These tools enable you to set personalized goals, track progress, and make informed adjustments. Mobile apps, such as MyFitnessPal and Strava, complement wearables by logging exercise routines and nutritional intake. They provide a platform to analyze trends and identify areas for improvement, allowing you to seamlessly tailor your approach to fitness and nutrition into your lifestyle (SOURCE 1).

Establishing baselines and setting goals are foundational to any health improvement plan. Conduct an initial fitness assessment to determine your current levels in key areas like strength, endurance, and flexibility. This assessment serves as a starting point, allowing you to set realistic, measurable goals using the SMART criteria: Specific, Measurable, Attainable, Relevant, and Time-bound. For instance, if your baseline reveals limited flexibility, aim to increase your range of motion by dedicating 15 minutes to stretching each day. As you progress, these goals can evolve, challenging you to reach new heights and stay motivated over the long term (SOURCE 4).

Regular health assessments are essential to measure progress and make necessary adjustments. Schedule periodic check-ups with healthcare providers to receive professional evaluations, ensuring that your practices align with your health needs. These assessments offer an opportunity to celebrate achievements and identify growth areas. Reviewing your progress every few months can instill a sense of accomplishment and reinvigorate your commitment to holistic health. Keeping a health journal or using digital tools to document milestones can provide valuable insights and encourage continued dedication to your well-being goals. By tracking these metrics, you can take control of your health journey, making informed decisions that promote a balanced and fulfilling lifestyle.

17.2 Emotional and Mental Health Metrics

Understanding your emotional and mental health is like having a compass. It guides you through daily life, helping you navigate challenges with resilience and clarity. Recognizing changes in mood and emotional stability over time provides insight into your mental well-being. You might notice patterns in how you react to stress or how your mood fluctuates throughout the day. These observations can reveal underlying issues that may need attention. Evaluating your stress levels and coping mechanisms is crucial. Stress, if left unchecked, can affect every aspect of life, from sleep to relationships. Consider whether you turn to healthy coping strategies, like exercise or talking to a friend, or if you rely on less constructive habits. Observing your mental clarity and focus during daily activities can also offer valuable clues. Do you find it difficult to concentrate at work? Are you easily distracted by thoughts? These may indicate stress or fatigue. Sleep quality and duration are strong indicators of mental health. Poor sleep can exacerbate anxiety and depression, creating a cycle that's hard to break. Monitoring these aspects can provide a comprehensive picture of your mental and emotional state.

Self-assessment tools can be valuable allies in this process. Mood tracking journals or apps allow you to reflect on your feelings daily. Recording your emotional responses to events can help you identify triggers and patterns over time. Stress scales and questionnaires can quantify your stress levels, offering a tangible measure of what might otherwise feel overwhelming. These tools can guide you in making informed decisions about your well-being. They can also serve as a record of your growth, showing how your emotional and mental health evolves.

Incorporating feedback from others can offer new perspectives on your well-being. Trusted friends or family members can provide insights into changes they observe, such as increased irritability or withdrawal. These observations can prompt self-reflection and encourage you to seek support if needed. Regular therapy or counseling sessions provide a safe space to explore your thoughts and emotions with a professional. Therapists can offer strategies to cope with stress and improve mental health, enhancing your self-awareness and resilience. Their guidance can be invaluable in navigating life's complexities, providing tools to foster emotional balance.

Setting specific goals for emotional and mental wellness can help you create a more balanced life. Establishing a meditation or mindfulness practice can enhance mental clarity and reduce stress, promoting a sense of calm. Even a few minutes of focused breathing or mindful observation can make a difference. Creating a bedtime routine can improve sleep quality, setting the stage for restful nights and energized days. Consider activities like reading, gentle stretching, or listening to calming music before bed. Planning regular social activities can boost mood and reduce feelings of isolation. Whether it's a weekly coffee date with a friend or joining a local club, these connections can enrich your life and offer support.

Approaching emotional and mental health with intention and care can transform your well-being. By identifying key indicators, utilizing self-assessment tools, seeking feedback, and setting goals, you can cultivate a life filled with clarity, resilience, and joy.

17.3 Spiritual Growth Indicators

In our fast-paced world, recognizing signs of spiritual growth can often be overlooked, yet they are deeply significant. As you cultivate a spiritual practice, you may notice an increased sense of peace and contentment in your daily life. This tranquility is not about the absence of challenges but rather a deeper acceptance of them. It's about finding calm amidst chaos, a steady center that anchors you. Alongside this inner peace, you might feel a greater empathy and compassion toward others. This shift is like opening a window to the world, where understanding and kindness flow more freely. It's an expansion of the heart, recognizing shared humanity and offering genuine care. Moreover, a strengthened connection to a higher purpose or meaning can emerge. This connection can manifest as a clear sense of direction or a newfound dedication to living in alignment with your values. It's a feeling that your actions, no matter how small, contribute to a larger tapestry of life, bringing you closer to a sense of fulfillment.

Self-reflection and spiritual journaling are powerful tools for fostering and tracking spiritual development. Writing about personal insights and shifts in perspective can illuminate the path you've traveled and reveal where you may wish to go. Through the act of journaling, you create a sacred space for introspection, where thoughts and feelings can be explored without judgment. Reflecting on experiences that foster spiritual awakening, whether it's a moment of awe in nature or a profound conversation, can deepen your understanding of your spiritual journey. These reflections can act as guideposts, reminding you of the growth you've experienced and the lessons learned. Spiritual diaries can also serve as a bridge between intention and action, helping you align your daily life with your spiritual aspirations. By putting pen to paper, you clarify your thoughts and intentions, making the abstract tangible and the journey more purposeful (SOURCE 3).

Engaging consistently with spiritual practices is vital for measuring growth. Whether through meditation, prayer, or religious rituals, these practices provide a framework for developing and nurturing your spiritual self. Regular participation offers a rhythm to your spiritual life, creating a foundation upon which deeper understanding can be built. Attending spiritual retreats or workshops can also enrich your practice, offering opportunities to learn from others and explore new perspectives. These immersive experiences can act as catalysts for growth, providing insight and inspiration that can be integrated into daily life. By engaging with these practices, you create a dialogue with your inner self, fostering a sense of connection and purpose that transcends the everyday.

Guidance and mentorship play a crucial role in spiritual growth. Connecting with spiritual mentors can provide support and direction, helping you navigate the complexities of your spiritual path. These mentors offer wisdom and experience, serving as both guides and companions on your journey. Participating in community discussions or study groups can also be invaluable. These gatherings offer a space for shared learning and reflection, where diverse perspectives can enrich your understanding. In these communities, you find not only support but also a sense of belonging, knowing that you're part of something larger than yourself. The insights gained from mentors and community can illuminate your path, offering clarity and encouragement as you continue to grow.

As you reflect on these indicators of spiritual growth, consider how they manifest in your life. Spiritual development is a deeply personal and transformative process, one that offers profound insights and a greater understanding of yourself and the world around you. By cultivating these practices and seeking guidance, you can nurture a more meaningful connection to your inner self and to the greater whole. Recognizing and embracing this growth is a step toward a more balanced and fulfilling life. As we conclude this chapter, remember that spiritual growth, like all aspects of holistic health, is an ongoing process. In the next chapter, we will explore how to sustain holistic health practices over the long term, ensuring that the insights and progress you've gained continue to enrich your life.

Chapter 18
Sustaining Holistic Health Long-Term

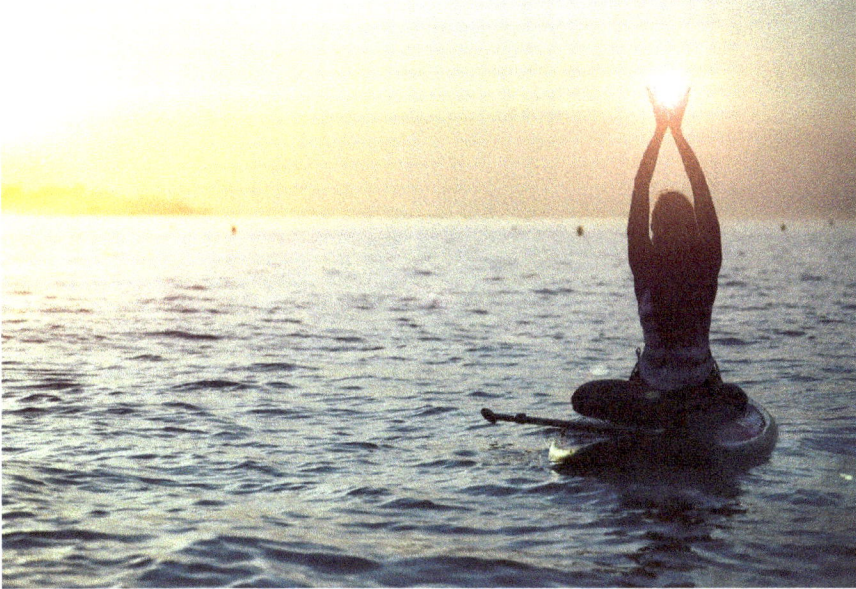

The sound of birdsong at dawn has always been a gentle reminder of nature's rhythm, a rhythm that is both constant and ever-changing. It was during one such morning, as I lay in bed contemplating the day ahead, that I realized how much this rhythm mirrored our own motivation cycles. Just as the sun rises and sets, our enthusiasm for holistic health practices can wax and wane. Understanding these natural fluctuations is crucial in maintaining long-term commitment to your well-being. Motivation is not a static force but a cycle influenced by diverse factors, including personal needs and external incentives (SOURCE 1). Recognizing the signs of declining motivation, such as procrastination or feelings of burnout, can prevent a downward spiral and encourage proactive measures. Conversely, identifying personal triggers that rekindle your drive, perhaps a motivational quote, a success story, or even the scent of fresh morning air, can help sustain your journey toward holistic health.

Setting long-term goals provides the direction and purpose needed to navigate this cyclical nature of motivation. Begin by envisioning your ultimate health aspirations, perhaps through a vision board filled with images and words that resonate with your desires. This tangible representation serves as a constant reminder of where you aim to be, keeping your goals alive in your mind. Break down these long-term visions into manageable, actionable short-term steps. This not only makes the process less daunting but also creates opportunities for regular achievement, each step a milestone on your path to wellness. Each short-term goal achieved fuels further motivation, reinforcing your commitment and providing momentum.

Variety and enjoyment are crucial in maintaining interest and enthusiasm in holistic practices. Imagine the monotony of eating the same meal every day or performing the same exercise routine without variation. The human spirit thrives on change and exploration. Consider trying new activities such as dance or martial arts, which not only enhance physical fitness but also stimulate the mind and spirit. Incorporate fun elements into your routines, perhaps music that uplifts your mood or outdoor settings that inspire a sense of adventure. This approach transforms your health practices from chores into enjoyable activities, making them something you eagerly anticipate rather than something you endure.

Accountability is another powerful tool in sustaining motivation and consistency in your holistic health journey. Partnering with a friend or mentor for regular check-ins creates a sense of obligation and support. This partnership can be as simple as a weekly phone call to discuss progress or challenges, providing both encouragement and accountability. Joining online groups or forums dedicated to holistic health allows you to share your journey with others who have similar goals. These communities offer a wealth of support, advice, and shared experiences, enriching your journey and keeping you connected and inspired.

Reflection Exercise: Motivation Mapping

Create a mind map that visually represents your motivation cycle. Start with your central goal in the middle and branch out with personal triggers, potential setbacks, and strategies for overcoming them. Include elements that inspire you and actions that have previously reignited your motivation. Keeping this map visible serves as a constant reminder of your journey, empowering you to navigate the ebbs and flows of motivation with intention and clarity.

18.1 Navigating Setbacks and Challenges

Life, with its unpredictable twists and turns, often presents challenges that can derail even our best-laid plans for holistic health. Amidst the daily hustle, it's not uncommon to find ourselves juggling multiple responsibilities, such as demanding work hours and family commitments. These time constraints can make it difficult to maintain a consistent routine of self-care and wellness practices. You may find that your planned meditation session is interrupted by a last-minute meeting, or your intention to prepare a healthy meal is compromised by a long commute. Recognizing these potential hurdles allows you to prepare strategies in advance, such as setting aside time in your calendar specifically for wellness or perhaps involving family members in your practices. Temporary loss of interest or burnout is another common setback on the path to wellness. Enthusiasm can wane, making it easy to slide back into old habits. This is a natural part of any long-term commitment, not a sign of failure but a signal to reassess and adjust.

Building resilience is crucial for overcoming these challenges and maintaining a holistic lifestyle. One effective strategy is practicing positive self-talk. By reframing negative thoughts into empowering ones, you can shift your mindset from defeat to determination. Instead of thinking, "I don't have time for this," consider, "I will make time because it's important." Engaging in stress-relief activities, such as creative expression through art or writing, can also serve as a powerful outlet. These activities allow you to process emotions in a healthy way, providing a sense of relief and clarity. Nature walks, with their inherent tranquility, offer another means of stress relief, fostering a connection with the natural world that can soothe and rejuvenate the spirit.

Setbacks, while challenging, are also rich with opportunities for growth and learning. They provide a chance to conduct self-reflection, to delve into the triggers and responses that led to the setback. By understanding these elements, you can gain valuable insights into your personal patterns and adjust your goals and strategies accordingly. Perhaps a particular practice isn't resonating with you anymore, or your schedule has changed, necessitating a different approach. Flexibility and adaptability are key here, allowing you to realign your path with your current needs and circumstances.

During these times, reaching out for support and resources can make a significant difference. Consult healthcare professionals who can provide guidance and reassurance during health setbacks. Their expertise can offer new perspectives and solutions you may not have considered. Additionally, community resources, such as local wellness centers or support groups, can provide encouragement and a sense of belonging. These groups offer the opportunity to connect with others who understand your challenges, fostering a supportive network that uplifts and inspires.

18.2 Evolving Your Holistic Health Journey

Life is a continuous ebb and flow, a series of transformations that shape who we are. In the realm of holistic health, embracing change is not just beneficial; it's vital. As you progress, you'll notice growth within yourself, subtle shifts that align with your evolving values and goals. Perhaps your initial focus was on physical fitness, but over time, you've developed an interest in mental well-being or spiritual exploration. These signs of transformation are natural markers of progress. They reflect your adaptability and willingness to grow beyond your current limits. It's essential to adapt your practices to align with these new aspirations. This might mean altering your exercise routine, incorporating new dietary habits, or embracing mindfulness practices that resonate with your current state of mind. Recognizing and welcoming these changes allows you to remain attuned to your inner needs, fostering a more fulfilling and authentic path.

Exploration is at the heart of holistic health. It's about expanding your repertoire and finding practices that resonate with you on a deeper level. Consider attending workshops or retreats where you can learn advanced techniques and immerse yourself in a supportive environment. These experiences offer insights and skills that can enhance your practice, providing tools to navigate life's complexities. Experimenting with alternative therapies like sound healing or aromatherapy can also open new avenues of healing. Sound healing uses the vibrations of instruments or the human voice to promote relaxation and emotional release, while aromatherapy employs essential oils to stimulate physical and psychological well-being. These therapies are not only innovative but also complementary to traditional practices, offering diverse approaches to nurturing your health.

Balancing tradition with innovation requires a thoughtful approach, one that respects the wisdom of the past while embracing the possibilities of the present. Modern wellness technologies, such as wearable fitness trackers or meditation apps, can enhance your holistic practices by providing real-time feedback and personalized recommendations. These tools, when integrated with time-tested methods, create a comprehensive practice that supports your overall well-being. However, it's important to evaluate new trends for alignment with your personal health philosophy. Not every innovation will suit your needs or resonate with your values. By maintaining a discerning eye, you can selectively incorporate advancements that genuinely enhance your practice, ensuring that they complement rather than overshadow traditional methods.

Documenting your experiences and progress is a valuable exercise in reflection and celebration. Keeping a holistic health journal allows you to capture achievements and insights, offering a tangible record of your journey. This practice not only tracks your growth but also provides clarity and motivation during challenging times. You might also consider creating multimedia records, such as photo diaries or video logs, to visually chronicle your transformation. These records serve as powerful reminders of your dedication and resilience, highlighting the milestones and moments of joy that have defined your path.

In the grand tapestry of life, your holistic health journey is a vibrant thread, weaving together change, exploration, and balance. By embracing growth, exploring new practices, and documenting your progress, you create a dynamic narrative that reflects your evolving self. This journey is not just about reaching a destination but about discovering and nurturing the many facets of your being, creating a life of harmony and fulfillment. As you continue to evolve, remember that each step forward is a testimony to your commitment and courage, guiding you toward a future rich with potential and well-being.

Conclusion

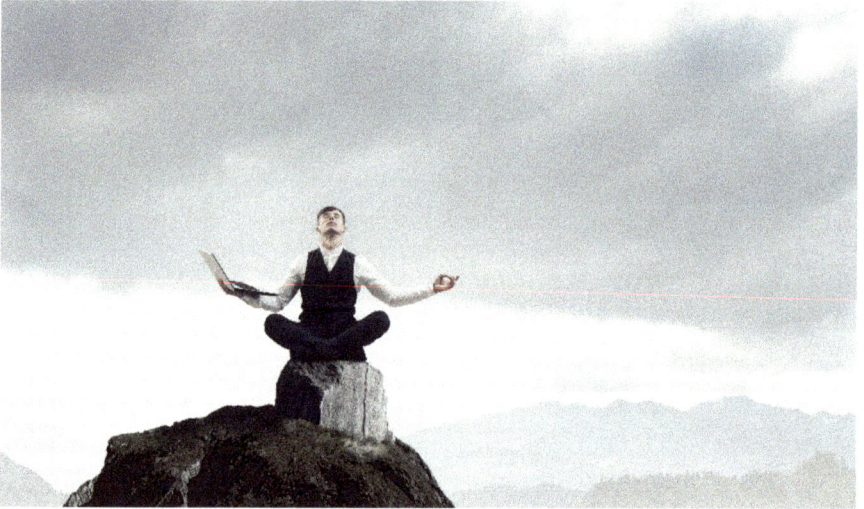

As we reach the end of this journey together, I hope you have come to appreciate the profound interconnectedness of mind, body, and spirit in achieving holistic health. Throughout this book, we've explored how integrating various practices into daily life leads to balanced living and inner peace. By embracing holistic health, you align yourself with a philosophy that honors every aspect of your being, paving a path toward true well-being.

Key takeaways from our exploration include the importance of personalized health plans and the value of emotional, mental, and spiritual wellness. You've discovered practical strategies to incorporate these elements into your life, from mindfulness meditations and balanced nutrition to exercise routines that fit seamlessly into a busy schedule. These practices are not mere additions to your routine but transformative tools that can reshape your life.

Reflecting on my own journey, I am reminded of the transformative power of holistic health. For over three decades, I have embraced these practices, which have profoundly enriched my life. They have taught me resilience, balance, and an ever-deepening connection to myself and the world around me. It is this personal transformation that I wish to share with you, knowing that you, too, can experience similar growth and fulfillment.

Now, you are empowered with the tools and knowledge to take control of your health. It begins with small, deliberate steps. Choose one or two practices that resonate with you and incorporate them into your routine. Be patient with yourself, and remember that change is a gradual process. As you grow more comfortable, expand your repertoire, and explore new dimensions of holistic health.

I urge you to begin your own holistic health journey today. The path is yours to take, and the time is now. Whether it's starting each day with a five-minute meditation or preparing a wholesome meal, taking that first step will set the foundation for a healthier, more fulfilling life.

For those looking to deepen their understanding, there are countless resources available. Books, websites, and community groups offer rich insights and support as you continue your exploration. Engage with these resources to enhance your journey and connect with others who share your aspirations.

I invite you to share your experiences and feedback. Your journey is unique, and your insights can inspire others. Connect with like-minded individuals through social media or other platforms. Join a community of holistic health enthusiasts, and together, we can foster a dialogue that encourages growth and transformation.

Looking ahead, I envision a future where holistic health becomes a mainstream approach to well-being. I hope for a world where balance, mindfulness, and interconnectedness are the norms, guiding us toward healthier lives. Holistic health is not static; it evolves and adapts to meet the needs of future generations. By embracing it, we contribute to a legacy of wellness that can inspire positive change for years to come.

Thank you for allowing me to be part of your journey. May you find joy, peace, and fulfillment as you step into the world of holistic health.

References

- Ayurveda and Traditional Chinese Medicine https://pmc.ncbi.nlm.nih.gov/articles/PMC1297513/
- Mind-body connection is built into the brain, study suggests https://new.nsf.gov/news/mind-body-connection-built-brain-study-suggests
- Mindfulness meditation: A research-proven way to reduce ... https://www.apa.org/topics/mindfulness/meditation
- Spiritual Wellness https://www.northwestern.edu/wellness/8-dimensions/spiritual-wellness.html
- The Power of Micro Meditation: Reducing Stress in Minutes https://sunnyhealthfitness.com/blogs/health-wellness/micro-meditation-reducing-stress?srsltid=AfmBOor6P8UBscIF0DJ1RTDIKHLsMce1eEdpLFrJAnZ8gvctxzTiwUyG
- 20 Meal-Prep Tips From People Who've Been Doing It For ... https://www.forksoverknives.com/how-tos/vegan-meal-prep-tips/
- 7 Benefits of High Intensity Interval Training (HIIT) https://www.healthline.com/nutrition/benefits-of-hiit
- The Best Fitness Apps for Busy People: Get Fit with Technology https://lifeisaproject.com/the-best-fitness-apps-for-busy-people-get-fit-with-technology/
- Processed vs. Whole Foods: The Science of Nutrition https://globalwellnessinstitute.org/global-wellness-institute-blog/2023/12/08/processed-vs-whole-foods-the-science-of-nutrition/
- A Guide to Holistic Nutrition Meal Plans https://theholistichighway.com/a-guide-to-holistic-nutrition-meal-plans/?srsltid=AfmBOoohdJ4s0T8hRXSEsinTgEQMLebqxHsa5UIHdbPmQFGkSrG-ozFd

- 16 Superfoods That Are Worthy of the Title
  https://www.healthline.com/nutrition/true-superfoods
- How to Incorporate Superfoods into Everyday Meals
  https://foodtolive.com/healthy-blog/how-to-incorporate-
  superfoods-into-everyday-
  meals/?srsltid=AfmBOoqESVsznr8Z_84yBR_JModdOfh5tsjwoY
  gSa8C2rFplqZVF2xJv
- Mindfulness Exercises by Jon Kabat-Zinn
  https://mbsrtraining.com/mindfulness-exercises-by-jon-kabat-
  zinn/
- 12 Science-Based Benefits of Meditation
  https://www.healthline.com/nutrition/12-benefits-of-meditation
- The Best Meditation Apps, Tried and Tested in 2024
  https://www.verywellmind.com/best-meditation-apps-4767322
- Mindfulness exercises https://www.mayoclinic.org/healthy-
  lifestyle/consumer-health/in-depth/mindfulness-exercises/art-
  20046356
- Herbal medicine Information | Mount Sinai - New York
  https://www.mountsinai.org/health-library/treatment/herbal-
  medicine#:~:text=What%20is%20the%20history%20of,as%20earl
  y%20as%203%2C000%20BC.
- Turmeric and Ginger: Combined Benefits and Uses - Healthline
  https://www.healthline.com/nutrition/turmeric-and-
  ginger#:~:text=Both%20turmeric%20and%20ginger%20can,doses
  %20of%20turmeric%20or%20ginger.
- How to Choose High Quality Herbs and Spices
  https://blog.mountainroseherbs.com/how-to-choose-the-best-
  herbs-and-spices
- Dilution Guidelines for Essential Oil Safety
  https://www.aromatics.com/blogs/wellness/dilution-guidelines-
  for-essential-oil-
  safety?srsltid=AfmBOoo46nTAHvC5R0ChJ7g_ADldgo3F7wC4fq
  eUvvBZ8qrRDmePaBL2

- How Yoga Affects the Brain and Body to Reduce Stress https://longevity.stanford.edu/lifestyle/2023/10/03/how-yoga-affects-the-brain-and-body-to-reduce-stress/#:~:text=Accordingly%2C%20yoga%20has%20been%20shown,of%20neurotransmitters%2C%20such%20as%20GABA.
- Hatha vs Yin Yoga: Understanding the Differences and Benefits https://mymeditatemate.com/blogs/yoga/hatha-vs-yin-yoga-differences-benefits-guide
- A sharper mind: tai chi can improve cognitive function https://www.health.harvard.edu/mind-and-mood/a-sharper-mind-tai-chi-can-improve-cognitive-function
- 8 Best Apps for Learning Tai Chi Using Your Smartphone https://www.makeuseof.com/apps-learning-tai-chi-using-smartphone/
- Creating Your Wellness Care Plan: Tips for Setting Health Goals https://www.purewellnesschiro.com/post/creating-your-wellness-care-plan-tips-for-setting-health-goals
- Holistic Self-Assessment https://www.aurorahealthcare.org/-/media/Project/Health-System-Enterprise/AuroraHealthCareOrg/aurorahealthcare/documents/services/integrative-medicine/holistic-self-assessment.pdf?rev=8aa636e1495046aaabdf9e0771321d9d&hash=A55F9A76993F9B506810982C9E614D64
- Effects of Healthy Lifestyles on Chronic Diseases: Diet, ... https://pmc.ncbi.nlm.nih.gov/articles/PMC10650398/
- SMART Goals: The Health Coaching Cheat Code https://functionalmedicinecoaching.org/blog/smart-goals/
- Cleaning Supplies and Household Chemicals https://www.lung.org/clean-air/indoor-air/indoor-air-pollutants/cleaning-supplies-household-chem
- 12 Natural Cleaning Recipes + Printable "Cheat Sheet" https://thenerdyfarmwife.com/natural-cleaning-recipes/

- NASA compiles list of best plants to clean indoor air
  https://www.co2meter.com/blogs/news/nasa-compiles-list-of-best-plants-to-clean-indoor-air?srsltid=AfmBOoqZSHriFsXqgqhC0kRCsm9vBM_FkPLcSaMBDIvrze2T13XM55-J

- Feng Shui Principles and Tips for Beginners
  https://www.thespruce.com/feng-shui-tips-for-beginners-1274536

- Physical Activity Benefits for Adults 65 or Older
  https://www.cdc.gov/physical-activity-basics/health-benefits/older-adults.html

- Cognitive Health and Older Adults | National Institute on Aging
  https://www.nia.nih.gov/health/brain-health/cognitive-health-and-older-adults

- 12 Best Superfoods for Older Adults
  https://health.usnews.com/wellness/food/slideshows/superfoods-for-older-adults

- The Importance of Staying Hydrated for Seniors
  https://www.aegisliving.com/resource-center/the-importance-of-staying-hydrated/

- Mental Health Benefits of Journaling
  https://www.webmd.com/mental-health/mental-health-benefits-of-journaling

- Social Support and Resilience to Stress
  https://pmc.ncbi.nlm.nih.gov/articles/PMC2921311/

- 8 Breathing Exercises for Anxiety You Can Try Right Now
  https://www.healthline.com/health/breathing-exercises-for-anxiety

- CBT Techniques: Tools for Cognitive Behavioral Therapy
  https://www.healthline.com/health/cbt-techniques

- Integrative Medicine: What Is It, Types, Risks & Benefits
  https://my.clevelandclinic.org/health/treatments/21683-integrative-medicine

- Talking With Your Doctor or Health Care Provider
  https://www.nih.gov/institutes-nih/nih-office-director/office-communications-public-liaison/clear-communication/talking-your-doctor
- Chronic Pain and Complementary Health Approaches
  https://www.nccih.nih.gov/health/chronic-pain-and-complementary-health-approaches-usefulness-and-safety
- Acupuncture: Effectiveness and Safety | NCCIH
  https://www.nccih.nih.gov/health/acupuncture-effectiveness-and-safety
- 18 Self-Care Tips for Busy People – Georgia HOPE
  https://gahope.org/18-self-care-tips-for-busy-people/
- Rethinking Rest
  https://www.mentalhealth.org.uk/sites/default/files/2022-06/Rethinking-Rest-guide-from-the-Mental-Health-Foundation.pdf
- 10 Ways to Build and Preserve Better Boundaries
  https://psychcentral.com/lib/10-way-to-build-and-preserve-better-boundaries
- 10 Apps to Help You Embrace Self-Care
  https://www.cnet.com/tech/services-and-software/10-apps-to-help-you-embrace-self-care/
- The Amazing Power of Online Wellness Communities - LinkedIn
  https://www.linkedin.com/pulse/amazing-power-online-wellness-communities-pauli-e--eqibe#:~:text=Wellness%20communities%20on%20the%20internet,passion%20for%20a%20healthy%20lifestyle.
- Examples of Successful Community-Based Public ...
  https://www.tfah.org/wp-content/uploads/2018/09/Examplesbystate1009.pdf
- The role of the family in health promotion: a scoping review ...
  https://pmc.ncbi.nlm.nih.gov/articles/PMC9673498/

- 9 Home Remedies Backed by Science
  https://www.healthline.com/health/home-remedies
- HelpGuide.org: Home https://www.helpguide.org/
- 28 Healthy Foods That Are Incredibly Cheap
  https://www.healthline.com/nutrition/29-cheap-healthy-foods
- Eat Healthy on a Budget: Plan Ahead
  https://www.heart.org/en/healthy-living/healthy-eating/eat-smart/nutrition-basics/eat-healthy-on-a-budget-by-planning-ahead
- Ayurvedic Medicine: An Introduction
  https://www.govinfo.gov/content/pkg/GOVPUB-HE20-PURL-gpo29672/pdf/GOVPUB-HE20-PURL-gpo29672.pdf
- Traditional Chinese Medicine: What You Need To Know
  https://www.nccih.nih.gov/health/traditional-chinese-medicine-what-you-need-to-know
- Ayurvedic Medicine: In Depth | NCCIH
  https://www.nccih.nih.gov/health/ayurvedic-medicine-in-depth
- Acupuncture in persons with an increased stress level— ...
  https://pmc.ncbi.nlm.nih.gov/articles/PMC7377446/
- Mindfulness meditation to control pain
  https://www.health.harvard.edu/pain/mindfulness-meditation-to-control-pain
- The role of acupuncture in the treatment of migraine - PMC
  https://pmc.ncbi.nlm.nih.gov/articles/PMC3291665/
- Herbs for Arthritis Pain Relief: Aloe Vera, Ginger, and More
  https://www.healthline.com/health/osteoarthritis/herbs-arthritis-pain
- 3 Holistic Approaches to Weight Loss: Inspiring Success ...
  https://bebeautyandhealth.com/holistic-approaches-to-weight-loss-in-cdm/
- Ultimate Comparison Of Top Activity Tracking Apps And ...
  https://www.hollyroser.com/post/ultimate-comparison-of-top-activity-tracking-apps-and-devices-for-peak-fitness/

- Meditation: A simple, fast way to reduce stress
  https://www.mayoclinic.org/tests-procedures/meditation/in-depth/meditation/art-20045858
- The Benefits of Spiritual Diaries: A Mixed-Method Study in Korea
  https://pmc.ncbi.nlm.nih.gov/articles/PMC8542544/#:~:text=Spiritual%20diaries%20can%20help%20participants,God%20(Yoo%2C%202017).
- 5 tips for setting realistic health goals
  https://www.peacehealth.org/healthy-you/5-tips-setting-realistic-health-goals
- The Motivation Cycle | Definition, Stages & Examples
  https://study.com/academy/lesson/the-motivational-cycle-definition-stages-examples.html
- Building Resilience with Holistic Wellness Strategies
  https://kimawellness.com/beyond-relief-building-resilience-with-holistic-wellness-strategies/
- The 5 Biggest Fitness and Wellness Technology Trends In ...
  https://bernardmarr.com/the-5-biggest-fitness-and-wellness-technology-trends-in-2023/
- The Benefits of Health Journaling: A Comprehensive Guide
  https://www.reflection.app/blog/the-benefits-of-health-journaling-a-comprehensive-guide

Share Your Thoughts – We Value Your Feedback!

Thank you for reading *Holistic Health: The Complete Guide to Balanced Living and Inner Peace*. I hope this book has inspired and empowered you to take meaningful steps toward a healthier and more harmonious life.

Your feedback is incredibly important, not only to me as the author but also to future readers who may be searching for guidance on their wellness journey. By sharing your thoughts, you help create a community of individuals dedicated to living a life of balance and vitality.

How You Can Help

If you enjoyed this book, learned something valuable, or found it transformative, I'd be truly grateful if you could take a few minutes to leave a review. Here's how:

1. Visit the platform where you purchased the book (Amazon, Goodreads, or other retailers).
2. Write a short review about your experience, what you loved, how it helped, or any insights you gained.
3. Share your story—your personal journey can inspire others to begin their path toward holistic health!

Suggestions for Your Review

- What part of the book resonated with you the most?
- Did you try any of the practices or tips mentioned?
- How has your perspective on health changed after reading the book?

Your honest review doesn't need to be long. Just a few sentences can make a big difference!

Stay Connected

If you'd like to share your feedback directly or ask questions, I'd love to hear from you. You can reach me at inobert007@gmail.com. Let's continue the conversation about aligning mind, body, and spirit!

With gratitude,
Dr. Inobert Pierre